Live Better Longer

Your Guide to a Healthier Life

Live Better Longer

Your Guide to a Healthier Life

by Hugh Wilson, M.D.

Monterey, California

May 2012

This book is an original work by Dr. Hugh Wilson. It taps into a long and successful professional career, and extensive research into the burgeoning new field of age management. All of the information is current. You are encouraged to visit the website LiveBetterLonger.info for explanatory graphics, new and updated information.

Live Better Longer
Your Guide to a Healthier Life

ISBN-10: 1475017774
ISBN-13: 978-1475017779

Printed in the United States of America

Table of Contents

Live Better Longer

Caveat Emptor

This is a medical information book, not a medical advice book. It is presented as an educational opportunity. It is not intended to diagnose or treat any disease or condition. The information provided in this book should not be construed as personal medical advice or instruction. No action should be taken based solely on the contents of this book. Do not disregard professional medical advice or delay seeking it because of something you have read in this book.

Readers should consult a physician or other appropriate health professionals on any matter relating to their health and well being.

The information and opinions provided here are believed to be accurate and sound, based on the best judgment available to the author, but readers who fail to consult appropriate health authorities assume the risk of any injuries. The author is not responsible for errors or omissions.

The author, editor and publisher shall not be held liable, nor be responsible to any person or entity with respect to any loss or damage caused, or alleged to be caused, directly or indirectly by the information contained in this book.

Live Better Longer

Dedication

To my son Andrew...
the greatest reason I can imagine
to Live Better Longer.

Live Better Longer

Publisher's Notes

When I first learned of the new direction that Hugh Wilson was taking with his medical background and knowledge, I knew that he was on an important new track. Our society is aging, and we aren't doing much to come to grips with the changes. For instance, we are now four generations alive at the same time, and the consequences of such an enormous social shift – and in a very short period of time – would be better assimilated with some serious, quality thinking in front of it.

That's why I urged Hugh to tell the story of aging from a physician's perspective. And not only because he has a medical background, but because he is a pioneer in the vital new field of age management. No, it's not about cosmetics – he's not writing about Botox or tummy tucks – but about the facts of how the body and the mind change as the years mount.

More important, he explains not only what happens to people as they age, but also what they can do to mitigate the normal processes inherent in aging. You should also be pleased to know that Hugh's approach is more about diet and exercise, rather than pharmacology, though he is perfectly conversant in all of the scientific issues involved in understanding the aging process.

This note...rather than use "he or she" and "him or her" throughout the book, a practice which while politically-correct tends to slow down the assimilation process, we chose to use just the masculine pronouns. Another reason is that men seem to be more stubborn about such issues as are discussed here, and it was thought they would feel more comfortable being addressed more directly.

A reminder, Age Management Medicine is a new field with many new discoveries as more people are drawn to it. A glossary has been included in the back of the book for your edification. Also, we will update the website as warranted, so please check in online at LiveBetterLonger.info.

Also, thank you to Denise Swenson, John Hayden, and Wes Lindberg for proofreading.

Tony Seton
April 2012

Introduction

The older I get, which I do deftly and with alacrity, the more truth I find in truisms. Despite the rapidity with which we accumulate new knowledge, some recurrent themes still often ring true. Like this from one of my favorite authors, Robert Heinlein: TANSTAAFL, which means There Ain't No Such Thing As A Free Lunch.

There's no free lunch when it comes to remaining healthy with age. It isn't as simple as taking a pill or eating the newest super food. And the hidden costs of apathy and denial will ultimately rear their ugly head. No, health requires effort. Intellectual and physical effort. It has to be understood and pursued.

This book is not intended as a scientific treatise or text but rather as an educational tool towards a better understanding of aging for seekers of better health. It won't meet the classroom needs of medical students or professors. But it is my fervent hope that it will motivate you to walk past the "free lunch" sign to find for yourself the tools to Live Better Longer.

Hugh Wilson, M.D.
Monterey, California

Live Better Longer

Why Living Longer...

Has a Downside

What Is Age Management?

When one speaks of getting old, it all comes down to this: "Aging is mandatory; debility is optional." In other words, our age is what it is today, and will be what it is five or ten or fifteen years from now. We can't change it. Those years go right by without stopping. They don't ask for our permission to pass Go and collect $200. They just go right on by without even a backwards glance over the shoulder. But let us remember that our age is just a number; it's how we feel that really matters.

My first recollection of being acutely, personally aware of the inexorable march of time was during a conversation with one of my older sisters, Katrina, when I was in my early twenties. She was contemplating a career change. She had gone to college to become a teacher. She had earned a bachelor's degree in education, and then her teaching credential, but she quickly learned that she didn't enjoy teaching and she decided to pursue another path.

During college, Katrina had worked part-time as a paralegal. Now at this later juncture in her life, she was discussing with a friend the possibility of attending law school. Katrina later related to me that she said to her friend, "But if I do this, I won't graduate until I'm forty." (Can't you hear her saying "forty" as though it was the end of the world?) To which my sister's friend replied most sagely, "Katrina, you're going to be forty with or without a law degree."

That was when it hit me. In your twenties, you're not typically focused on or struck by the thought of being forty. It was a fantasy world our parents told us about when they were in their forties, but we never really believed in it. Believed? Heck we didn't even stop to consider being forty! Not only didn't we believe, but we scoffed at the very notion. It was surely just so much more parental gobbledygook.

But the reality is, of course, that most of us are going to be forty and fifty and eighty, and our arrival at these hallmarks is just a matter of pages pulled inexorably off of the calendar. And we will reach that age with or without good health. The process is going to happen to us with or without our consent or even recognition. What I mean is, we can't see ourselves grow incrementally minute by minute, or even day by day.

So whether we find it upsetting or amusing, we must resign ourselves to the fact that we're all going to age. It's better than the alternative.

The central concept of Age Management is about how we can turn that process to our best advantage. To age as well as we can, instead of letting age happen to us. If there's anything that we can do actively to improve the process, that's called Age Management. (I prefer to call it *Living Better Longer*, as you will see in the coming pages.)

Age Management is an effort to make the best of your health as you age, rather than bemoaning the number of candles on your birthday cake. We are going to reach that age, whichever it is that concerns us. Maybe our hair is creeping back on our forehead, or parts of us that used to be firm seem droopy. The specific number isn't as important as our real-life actual health. Age Management teaches us how we can live with our age better, and as best as we can. The choice, simply, is that we can let age happen to us or we can work with it, manage it, and make it work to our advantage.

I'm not talking about cosmetics. This isn't about Botox or plastic surgery where the packaging is pretty'd up while the inside corrodes.

You will learn in this book that Age Management is a new, science-based medical specialty with a proactive approach to optimizing human function and the quality of life. The goal is to mitigate the effects of aging prior to the onset of degenerative disease processes, and to chart a new course so that you can remain vital, and minimize your risk of getting age-related diseases. Though aging cannot be stopped, Age Management can help extend your health span - the period of one's life during which we are generally healthy and free from serious or chronic illness - and help you live healthier, longer, and better.

The History of Age Management

The original term to describe the concept of promoting prolonged good health was "anti-aging." The effort to establish this as a new medical specialty began in the 1980s. It was at a time when the scientific community had recorded an historic hundred years of almost immeasurable gains in human health and longevity. The average American Caucasian woman born in 1850 could expect to live approximately forty years. By 1980 that number was nearly eighty. How did that happen?

Most of the severe acute illnesses that had accounted for a majority of deaths throughout history until the latter part of the 19th century – the epidemic infectious diseases – were no longer a significant threat to Western society. I'm speaking here of the average person living in North America and western Europe. This was due to such literally life-changing developments of late the 19th and early 20th centuries as the building of effective sewage systems that curbed and then prevented waterborne epidemics. Also, scientists and physicians discovered vaccines that could prevent many other viral and bacterial infections. And then came the antibiotics which enabled the treatment of those bacterial infections that weren't prevented.

It was when these massive killers were unmasked and dealt with that it was revealed what problems were less the result of the social environment and more due to what we thought of at the time as simple aging. What was left were the chronic degenerative and inflammatory diseases that had not been especially apparent previously – before so many people were living longer – and which were not treatable on a public level; they required individual treatment. This approach to finding health solutions for normal issues that are part of aging became the foundation upon which Age Management Medicine (AMM) was built.

Keep it Clean

Evidence of early forms of sanitary sewage conveyance – or sewer systems in the vernacular – date back to the Minoan city of Knossos four millennia before the birth of Christ. And as far back as 800 BC, the Romans used a combination of aqueducts and sewers to separate fresh water and waste. These technologies were largely lost though during the dark ages and the modern day equivalent of what we now recognize as waste water systems didn't come into being on any significant scale until centuries later. In fact, large scale planned and successful urban sewage systems did not become the norm in the Western Hemisphere until the late 19th century.

Dysentery was the scourge of 19th century armies where

men lived in close quarters with poor sanitation. It was years after the Civil War that numerous urban dwellers still used unreliable "privies" and cesspools. Epidemics of cholera and typhoid were known threats up to that time in major U.S. cities. Columbus, Ohio, was hit by cholera in 1833, and New York City the following year. There were cholera outbreaks in London in 1848 and 1854, with tens of thousands of people falling ill, and many of them dying. The Union Army lost as many as 80,000 men to typhoid during the War between the States. Chicago experienced a typhoid epidemic in 1891.

When finally in place, successful sewage operations were a huge first step in prolonging human life. So keeping fresh water and waste water separate may well have been the greatest public health success in history. It largely eliminated the scourge of water-borne infectious diseases. In the under-developed world today, where good sewage is still not yet the norm, the leading cause of death in children is dehydration, secondary to diarrhea caused by water-borne infections. We just don't see that in the developed world any more.

Shot of Prevention

The large scale development and distribution of vaccines followed close on the heels of the development of urban sewage. Vaccine research began, curiously enough, during the Dark Ages – probably around the end of the first millennium – but it didn't begin to get fully underway until the late 18th century. In 1796 Edward Jenner successfully prevented small pox in a young boy by first inoculating him with cow pox material.

There is an important distinction to be made regarding immunization – it happens both passively and actively. Passive immunization is the transfer of infection-fighting capability from a previously-infected person to a non-infected or recently exposed individual.

This is why it works. Among our basic human responses to infection are antibodies, which are large molecules made by immune cells that help kill infectious invaders. The ability to produce those same antibody molecules again in the future – if and when needed – continues for many years; in some instances, even a lifetime.

These antibodies – and the cells that make them – circulate in the blood and so can be collected by drawing blood. Then the antibodies can be isolated from the other blood components and injected into a person, providing short-lived immunity. This is still the first step in treating persons who have been exposed to rabies. Other than rabies, use of passive immunization is now the exception rather than the norm.

In active immunization, instead of giving a person antibodies, they are given molecular fragments of the particular viruses or bacteria. These fragments are either completely inactive (killed) virus, or weakened (attenuated) virus. The latter weakened versions are considered "live" viruses. In such active immunizations, the recipient gets a much milder version of the disease, and his immune system produces antibodies to combat the invader, so as to prevent further susceptibility, all without the patient becoming dangerously or even seriously ill. It's certainly better to suffer some flu-like symptoms for a day or so than to deal with a major disease that could even be life-threatening.

By the late 19th century, first efforts at rabies vaccination were underway. The earliest version of Louis Pasteur's rabies vaccine came along in 1885. Jonas Salk's polio vaccine was introduced in the 1950s. By the mid 20th century, large scale vaccination programs were undertaken, and they soon became standard in the Western world. By the 1960s American children were routinely vaccinated against polio and small pox, and later came vaccinations for measles, mumps, German measles, whooping cough and tetanus, among others. The so-called common childhood illnesses became largely a thing of the past. While successful sewage systems saved us from water born infections, vaccines now protected us from infectious diseases with other modes of transmission.

Miracle Drug

After Louis Pasteur first proposed his germ theory of disease transmission in the mid-1800s, the search for compounds capable of killing microorganisms, without harming the host, began in earnest. Although there are unpublished accounts of "primitive" peoples using molds to treat would-be infections thousands of years earlier, penicillin is widely considered the first true antibiotic. It was discovered in 1928 when the Scottish scientist Alexander Fleming discovered in his laboratory that contaminants of the Penicillium mold species were hampering his efforts to grow the bacterium, staphylococcus aureus, in culture plates. By the early 1940s, penicillin was in widespread production and use. Not only were innumerable lives saved directly through its use in the treatment of life-threatening infections, but cases of post-infectious complications like rheumatic heart or kidney disease fell dramatically as well.

Sulfa antibiotics were first discovered in the 1930s. Early forms though were not readily absorbed in the intestinal tract. First attempts to manufacture oral sulfa preparations resulted in widespread toxicity including kidney failure and death, and thus early sulfas were confined to a role as topical treatments. (These early sulfa deaths are what prompted the formation of the U.S. Food and Drug Administration.) By the early 1940s though, sulfa drugs were in widespread use. During the Second World War, every American foot soldier, not just those in the medical corps, carried packets of crystalline sulfa antibiotic powder to help treat battle wounds.

New Problems

So in little more than seventy-five years, from roughly 1875 to 1950, modern science in the Western world had essentially eliminated water-born disease outbreaks, prevented numerous viral and bacterial illnesses, and had provided mechanisms for treating numerous life-threatening bacterial infections. Life spans increased dramatically in parallel with these advancements.

With these enormous advances in health care, by the mid-20th century, medical scientists were able to turn their research more toward the now more common non-infectious killers such as heart attack, stroke, and cancer; these being the new major causes of death for the longer-living population.

Concurrent with the decreasing death rate from infectious diseases, the 20th century saw a steady increase in the incidence of and death from cardio-vascular disease and stroke. Men and women who might previously have died an infectious death as a child, or as a young adult in their twenties and thirties, were now dying in their fifties of heart attacks and strokes. In 1948 an ambitious, large-scale epidemiologic study of cardiovascular disease was undertaken in

Framingham, Massachusetts by the National Heart Lung and Blood Institute and by Boston University. The researchers recruited over 5,000 men and women between the ages of thirty and sixty-two, and began the first round of extensive physical examinations and lifestyle interviews that were later analyzed for common patterns related to cardiovascular disease (CVD). The study led to the identification of the major CVD risk factors that are familiar to us today, i.e., high blood pressure, high blood cholesterol, smoking, obesity, diabetes, and physical inactivity. The study also revealed a great deal of valuable information on the effects of related factors such as blood triglyceride and HDL cholesterol levels, age, gender, and psycho-social issues, which in turn led to the public health efforts we are all so familiar with today.

The Big C

Though cancer has been recognized for centuries, the first diagnostic techniques for it came into being in the - you guessed it - mid-19th century. Along with new diagnostic procedures to visually explore body spaces like the esophagus, cervix, colon and bladder – directly or indirectly without surgery – there also came the use of the microscope to examine malignant cells in specimens obtained with those instruments.

Normal benign cells respect their neighbors. They grow and reproduce to within their normal boundaries but do not invade surrounding tissues. Malignant cells respect no boundaries. They invade surrounding tissues and also leave their site of origin by getting into tissue fluid or blood. This way they can travel to a new locations within the body, distant from their primary site of origin, and there they can not only survive, but also set up camp in new sites where they will continue to grow. This process is called metastasis.

This is why early detection is so important, and why early diagnosis has always been the mainstay of cancer care. Cancer in its early stages is typically confined to its primary site of origin. It hasn't yet spread to distant sites. Early diagnosis allows local therapy, most often surgical excision but sometimes, localized radiation therapy. This is a relatively recent development though; in the early days, little safe and effective therapy was known, let alone available.

Surgical excisions, using ether as anesthesia, began in the 1840s. Few in medicine at the time had proposed – and fewer still accepted – the germ theory of disease, and the rate of post-surgical infections was substantial. By the late 1860s, operative cleanliness was promoted and eventually became the norm. With that major development – you've certainly heard the phrase, cleanliness is next to godliness – surgical therapy made the leap from the experimental to the practical, and concomitantly validated the importance of early cancer detection.

A localized cancer could be entirely excised and cured.

But advanced cancers still thwarted the surgeon's best efforts. Once cancer has spread, it is no longer localized but has become systemic. Systemic disease requires systemic therapy; surgery is, of course, a local response.

The conceptual basis for chemotherapy is a chemical agent able to selectively kill malignant cells while ignoring normal, benign cells. The ideal chemo-therapeutic agent – analogous to antibiotics with bacteria – would kill 100% of malignant cells and no normal cells at all. Unfortunately, no such medication has been discovered as of the first decade of the 21st century. Nearly all chemotherapeutic agents are en-tirely non-specific, meaning that they will adversely affect every cell in some way.

The drugs are designed to interfere with the repro-ductive cycle of cells. Infused into the blood, the drugs circulate and have access to every cell in the body. Normal cells and cancer cells are equally exposed. But since malignant cell populations are on average replicating more than normal cells, they are harmed to a greater degree.

But it is only a matter of degree. Chemotherapy is a shotgun poison that hurts malignant and benign cells alike. That's why some people suffer so greatly from chemotherapy; their healthy cells are being destroyed along with the bad.

Another troublesome aspect to chemo is that the normal cells that are most affected are those with a high replication rate. Those are the blood-forming cells in marrow, lining cells of the gastrointestinal tract, and hair follicle cells. That is why chemotherapy patients often become anemic, suffer nausea, and lose their hair.

With all this improvement in the science and technique of treating cancer, the five-year relative survival rate for all cancers diagnosed between 1999 and 2006 is 68%, a whopping third higher from 50% in 1975-1977.

You have to be careful with statistics though. For instance, U.S. cancer death rates from 1950 to 2000 have increased by 2%. But the important fact behind that statistic is that all of the increase has been in older age people, and that's because we are living so much longer than we did in 1950. We are living long enough for the diseases of aging to become more prominent, and chief among them is cancer.

Success...Next?

The above successes resulted in dramatic increases in average life expectancy. As stated before, a Caucasian woman born in 1850 would, on average, expect to live to the age of 40.5. By 1900 that number was 51. By 1970 it was an astounding 75½. By 1980, just ten years later, it had reached 78¼. These advances represent a significant improvement, but also a substantial leveling off. [Different data sets show slightly varying results because there is no single definitive database for the entire United States – i.e., males and females and all ethnic groups – but the important point to note here is the dramatic trend.]

It was within this context of a remarkable steady increase in average expected life span, and a massively-improved quality of life occurring in less than 150 years, that the idea of individuals actively taking control of their own health – rather than relying solely on public health improvements and the directives of insurance companies – came into being. Physicians and patients alike began to see their health this way: "I've gotten my vaccinations, I take my high blood pressure medication, I go on walks, and I stopped eating at fast food restaurants. What more can I do?" Thus was born the anti-aging movement.

What You Should Know

Anti-Aging

In its short lifetime, anti-aging medicine has already taken a few turns and encountered interesting forks in the road. In basic terms, those working on anti-aging issues break into three groups. One group is comprised of researchers and doctors whose primary focus is to use cutting edge technology to prolong life. They've looked at the longest known living human ever, who was 122 years, and asked the question, "Why can't everyone live that long?"

These doctors are particularly interested in the latest - and still largely unproven therapies - like stem cell treatments, lengthening telomeres (more on this later) and nano-technologies. This latter is a broad science but the majorities of efforts are directed at synthetic drug delivery systems to bring very high concentrations of medication directly and specifically to the diseased site rather than distribute the drug systemically. In other words, to more accurately target the cells that need attention, instead of affecting the whole body. The concept, of course, is to bring more effective doses to bear where needed while preventing side effects elsewhere. This is an exciting concept but still highly experimental.

The second group of anti-aging doctors is focused on

improving appearances. They have been working to perfect approaches that will produce a more youthful look. Though these doctors use the term anti-aging, it would probably be more accurate to refer to them as cosmetic physicians. Some are surgeons but most provide injections of various fillers and Botox to change the contour of wrinkled faces. Many also recommend stem cell treatments.

The third group, the one I consider myself to be a member of, are those professionals who are focused on bringing current technology to bear not on appearance, but on actual health. While not ignoring longevity, we look principally at improving the quality of life and thus extending the health span. Our principal defining characteristic is not a new magical scientific discovery by scientists but rather a dedication to changing attitudes by the patient. We thoroughly reject the notion that people have no choice but to simply accept the changes of aging and that nothing can be done. We also discard the notion, "If it hurts, don't do it." Our bottom line is that quality of life can remain high as age rises, and not decline as used to be thought of as an inevitable outcome to growing older.

I don't wish to in any way denigrate my primary care medicine colleagues who are not involved in – or who in fact forsake – the concept and practice of anti-aging medicine. These are good people who are an essential component of the framework of modern Western medical care. Without them, AMM could not exist. I strongly recommend to all my patients that they maintain a relationship with their primary care provider to manage any chronic illnesses already acquired.

But the world of the primary care provider is concentrated on - and this may sound a bit cliché but it is entirely correct - diagnosis and treatment of disease rather than promoting health. The first thing a physician writes on his chart during a patient visit is the patient's "chief complaint." The physician then focuses his treatment in response to that "chief complaint." The primary care physician's process is totally complaint-driven, and his goal is to come up with an appropriate response to that complaint. Different responses may be tried, and further testing required, but the end goal of this facet of medicine is to produce an effective response to the patient's complaint. I should add that almost exclusively, the adjusted response will be a new prescription or a modification to an existing one.

Those complaints that don't lend themselves to a specific diagnosis within the "standard of care" – and invariably linked with the recommended prescription – are often just chalked up as complaints merely the result of getting older. This is particularly true, of course, with older patients, but not infrequently people in their forties will be told that they are not as young as they used to be.

And the recommendation is to learn to live with it. If doing something causes pain – like playing hard – don't do it; don't play hard. If you find yourself tired more often, get more sleep. If you don't sleep well, here's a prescription for a sedative. If you are unable to have sex anymore, try Viagra, and if that doesn't work for you, well, just learn to live with it because that's the way it is for older folks.

And there's this. If you want a more definitive discussion with your physician, "Sorry, he's in an HMO, and he can't spend any more time with you. However, you can see his nurse or assistant – for about six minutes, but that's about all the time available."

Now, again, please don't misunderstand. I am a believer in pharmacotherapeutics. I certainly write prescriptions for my patients **when appropriate for promoting health and longevity**. Pharmaceutical research, e.g. the development of vaccines and antibiotics as noted above, plus cholesterol and blood pressure medications, has been a driving force behind the extension of the human life span.

But we should also remember that every drug has unintended – and often undesirable – side effects, depending on the dose and the patient. Every drug combination carries risk for adverse reactions. And I'm not just talking of unpleasant consequences. In the journal *Pharmacological Reviews* (June 2004), authors Allan J. McLean and David G. Le Couteur reported that in older persons, "It has been estimated that adverse drug reactions are the fourth to sixth greatest causes of death, and approximately 5% to 10% of hospital admissions are related to the management of people suffering from drug-related toxicity." They also wrote that, "When adverse drug reactions occur in older people, they are more likely to be severe and less likely to be recognized or reported by the patient....This trend also has been observed in general practice...." E. R. Hajar and others concluded in the journal *American Journal of Geriatric Pharmacotherapeutics* in 2007 "that polypharmacy **continues to increase** (emphasis added) and is a known risk factor for important morbidity and mortality." (Polypharmacy is the use of multiple drugs.)

Concerned about the dangers of over-medication, to the maximum extent possible, AMM physicians rely instead on lifestyle modification, dietary supplements, and stress reduction. We make time to explore all of our patient's concerns, hopes, and especially goals, not just their current "complaints."

I am reminded of my medical school professors who encouraged me to "listen to your patients. They will tell you what's wrong." The point was two-fold. First, the professors were saying that we doctors shouldn't rely so heavily on radiographic and laboratory technology that we allow ourselves to miss significant diagnostic information offered directly by our patient's description of his concerns. Second, we should keep in mind that our patient's agenda may not be the same as ours. Don't forget to address your patient's agenda, they said.

In the classic film, *My Dinner with André*, there's a scene where the main character is with his father at the hospital, about to visit his desperately-ill mother. She is very ill and almost gone. One of her doctors on his rounds entered her room while the father and son waited in the hallway. When he came out he smilingly proclaimed to the grieving husband and son, "Isn't it great how well her arm is healing?" A lesion was healing on the arm of a dying woman. This was a perfect example of a doctor who was focused on the wrong agenda.

Perhaps the central tenet of Age Management is to reject the notion that all of the changes of aging are inevitable. While not ignoring patient complaints, the emphasis in Age Management is not on specific individual complaints, but on the whole process of change, and how we physicians can give our patients the tools they need to modulate their individual aging process. With objective metrics of body composition, fitness and hormonal status (details to follow), we can provide our patients with personalized dietary plans and fitness techniques that will improve their well being. Meanwhile, we can supplement their efforts with a more youthful hormonal balance specifically tailored to their individual condition, which then symbiotically enables them to achieve even greater benefits from their own efforts. More on that later.

The Insurance Factor

Along with the shift in consciousness that rejects the idea that aging is inevitably debilitating, there should be a willingness by both the physician and patient to take a further step. It's a big one. It means stepping outside the health insurance model that has dominated the practice of medicine in America for more than half a century.

The original concept of health insurance was as a backstop to prevent financial catastrophe in the event of medical catastrophe. It was not intended as a prospective payment plan for any and all medical expenses, no matter how small or routine, as we have now. The current insurance model is in lockstep with the complaint-response approach to health care, which means that it doesn't fit the changing needs of our aging population. So the insurance model is inappropriate for the growing number of people who don't believe in the inevitability of the debility of aging, and who are ready and willing to take responsibility for their own better health.

Some history on our insurance problem. The idea of "accident insurance" – which functions much as modern disability insurance does today – was available beginning as early as the late 19th century. And private health insurance to cover costs of hospitalization began only eighty years ago in the U.S.. It was still in its infancy in the 1940s when the Second World War broke out.

During the war, a high proportion of America's young men (and to a lesser extent women) were serving in the armed forces. There was intense competition at home for the labor services of the remaining men and women. To curb the resulting inflation, the Roosevelt administration imposed wage and price controls preventing employers from offering higher wages to attract the best employees.

But benefits were not controlled and so many employers began to offer health insurance benefits as an added incentive. Thus began the employer-provided health insurance system still in place today. Though not without its limitations, the system has worked fairly well for the majority of Americans; that is, until recently.

When health insurance was initially instituted, there was no heart bypass surgery and no arterial stents. Organ transplant technology had not yet been developed. There were only a limited number of antibiotics and no blood pressure or cholesterol-lowering medications. Computed tomography (CT scan) and magnetic resonance imaging (MRI) hadn't yet been imagined. There were essentially no chemotherapy drugs.

An American man born in 1941 could expect to live about sixty-three years. By 1965 when Medicare went into effect that number was sixty-eight. And by 2011 it was up to seventy-six. We now live about thirteen years longer, with far more abundant high-tech diagnostic and therapeutic tools. That is thirteen more years of health care to be provided that wasn't required when employer-funded plans began, and at a much more expensive rate to boot. Planning for these eventualities was not adequately considered in those early days. But then again, who could have foreseen all this progress?

The discussions on how to improve the system are many and varied. The bottom line though, is that at present, it is what we have and what we have to deal with.

Unlike most private business transactions in our society – where the company providing the product or service and the customer have a direct relationship with one another – in the modern American health care system, the majority of patients doesn't pay either their doctor or their insurance company. Instead, it's the patient's employer who pays the insurance company who then pays the physician. These are two enormous edifices between the patient and his doctor, and vice versa. (For the sake of a simplified explanation, I am leaving out co-pays and deductibles and am referring here only to premiums.)

The employer and the insurance company both have a stake in the financial specifics of the transaction; the former want to keep the price low, and the latter want to keep the price high. The employer decides how extensive a policy it is willing to purchase for its employee, and the insurance company then limits the patient's access to services accordingly. The insurance company also limits the doctor's access to reimbursement. Doctors spend considerable resources in personnel and time trying to get what they consider reasonable payment for the services they provide their patients, with the insurance companies obstructing and delaying the payment process wherever they deem such action cost-effective.

Obviously, and tragically, these are enormous obstacles to doctor-patient relationships. The fact is that in order for health care provider and consumer to re-establish a natural – let us say healthy – relationship, it is essential that they both agree to move outside of the insurance industry mandates. This not only reduces costs, but it also – and more importantly – improves the communications between doctor and patient, and thus enhances treatment. The patient is healthier, and both he and his doctor are happier.

Since much if not most of the services provided by Age Management physicians are not covered by the majority of insurance plans, AMM doctors seldom accept insurance. I will get into the specifics in greater detail in a subsequent chapter, but here is just one important example. It has to do with one of the most significant problems associated with aging and that is loss of muscle mass which contributes to frailty, falls, and lost independence; to name just a few consequences. The diagnostic term is sarcopenia, meaning diminished muscle.

Here's the rub, so to speak. In order for a healthcare provider to be paid for his services, the insurance company for any service requires the doctor to provide a specific diagnosis, and also a specific procedure that has been provided to the patient. The procedures have to be pre-approved for the diagnosis. The insurance industry has a list of diagnostic codes that has been established to standardize terminology. These are the International Classification of Disease, Ninth edition codes, referred to as ICD-9 codes. (They are soon to be revised to the ICD-10 codes). A complementary list of standardized procedural terminology is called the Current Procedural Terminology or CPT codes. The insurance industry has established which CPT codes are acceptable to pay any given ICD-9 code. If the diagnosis correlates to the procedure – if the ICD and CPT match up – the insurance company will pay the physician. If the codes don't match up, sorry, but no payment. At least not without a lengthy dispute.

Why is this is a particular problem for AMM work? Because in AMM we are usually starting without a particular complaint. Plus we are looking at the larger picture of health. Procedures are performed without a diagnosis to determine a patient's health; for instance, the muscle testing required to determine if sarcopenia is present. But to repeat, since there is no complaint per se, there can't be a formulaic (CPT) response. And so the insurance companies refuse to pay. In this way, the insurance industry limits patient's access to services, and the company's costs. Physicians can offer pro bono service to some needy individuals but obviously it is impossible to have a practice based entirely on performing their work for free.

For the moment, the choice is for the patient and the health care provider to do what needs to be done without the insurance net. The doctor and the patient will be in control of the process and the outcome. That will mean some up-front costs, but in the long run, there will be considerable health savings as conditions are perceived and responses developed. And most important, the patient will live better longer.

My Personal Journey to AMM

There is a sizeable number of physicians practicing Age Management Medicine, at centers around the country. I had seen their ads and was intrigued by their message. But my introduction to AMM was quite personal. It came via my experience as a patient.

I was fifty years old. I had always been active and enjoyed being active, but I was having more and more difficulty remaining active due to an increasing frequency of soft tissue injuries and general aches and pains. I was willing, at some level, to accept a diminished level of functionality. Like most everyone else, that's what I expected with age. But I wasn't willing to accept a steeply diminished level as seemed to be called for with my physical angst.

I wasn't being stubborn. My active lifestyle dated back to my youth. I began cycling as a means of conveyance at about twelve years old. When I began junior high school in the Los Angeles Unified School System in the 1960s, our home was several miles from my new school, and my mother worked. So guess what? On the bike I hopped, and it turned out that I enjoyed it. The freedom was liberating. By eighth grade I was taking distance rides for fun. A friend and I even planned a bicycle trip to San Diego that would have required an overnight stay but our parents would have none of that at our age. We did, however, make more than one round trip of about fifty miles to the beach at Santa Monica.

Later, I took an interest in backpacking. I had a backpack before I had a car, which was unusual in those days for my age group and my peers. Our parents would drive my friends Gary and Pat and me up to a trail head in the Angeles National Forest, drop us off and wish us the best of luck. We kissed the city life goodbye for a few splendid days at a time doing what we called boulder-hopping. We would often hike many miles off-trail, carrying everything we needed - food, water, shelter - on our backs. The folks would return in two or three days to find a group of hungry, dirty teenagers ready for a hot meal and a soft bed. (Can you imagine that in modern America?)

In junior high and high school I played football and that kept me in shape. Nothing like "two-a-days" - those twice-daily heavy practice sessions invented by high school football coaches to torture young would-be stars - to slim a guy down and build endurance. In college I took up running, surfing, and skiing. During medical school and internship there wasn't time for much, but I did manage to keep fit with an occasional run or bike ride. During residency and on into my thirties, I returned to cycling, both on and off road. I even took up off-road adventure racing - kayak, run, and bike - with my nephew Rob.

By my forties though, all of this physical activity left me with numerous, recurrent soft tissue injuries. I also found my energy/motivation for it was wearing down. So there were two issues. First, that I missed not doing as much as I used to. Second, that I wasn't quite as energetic about it as I once had been. And even when I felt the urge to get some exercise, I was often thwarted by pain or weakness. On those occasions when I had sufficient motivation and less pain, I noticed my performance declining and that was not only frustrating but disturbing.

So, in the fall of 2009, I contacted one of the nation's leading Age Management medical groups to see if there was anything they could do for me. The response was more than encouraging; they said, "We think we can help you, and we think that, if this works for you, you might like to become one of our doctors. We just so happen to have a training program in Age Management Medicine." They have multiple centers around the country, including Las Vegas, which is relatively convenient to Monterey.

I got a real education there. I learned about the hormonal and physiologic changes of aging and why I was having difficulty maintaining the same sort of energy/activity level that I had in the past. Most importantly, I learned that an age-related decline in energy levels was not inevitable, and what could be done about it. That intrigued me. Although I had always prided myself on my knowledge of nutrition and exercise physiology, I hadn't realized how much those fields had advanced over the years. I wasn't quite as knowledgeable as I had thought.

A few years ago at this writing, I had been a pathologist for over twenty years at that point. I was practicing surgical pathology and laboratory medicine, not forensics. In other words, I was using laboratory techniques to diagnose disease, the majority of them being cancer and infectious diseases. Not exclusively, but those were the entities that occupied the majority of my time and attention.

After my internship in internal medicine, I had always been involved in the diagnostic end of medicine, rather than the therapeutic side. But the older I became, the more I needed to understand therapy, and, synchronistically, the more interested I became in therapeutics. Physician, heal thyself! as the saying goes.

And there was another factor that was moving me toward a change. I didn't see a lot of patients as a pathologist, and I realized that I was missing that sense of personal contact. To some extent, I'd see patients as a consultant. As a pathologist, I served as a consultant to other doctors, which involved, sometimes, seeing their patients. But usually it was just for one visit. Plus it was usually patients who were hospitalized. Or occasionally I would be asked to stop by the offices of doctors which were within walking distance of the hospital, when they had a patient in their office whom they might want me to see.

I had partners in my pathology practice, and we had our own office where we also would see patients for procedures such as a bone marrow biopsy or a fine-needle aspiration biopsy. So, yes, just to be clear, as a pathologist I did see patients, but principally for a one-time consultation. It wasn't something that I'd typically do all day, every day. My work was primarily in the laboratory. Patient consultations were maybe a few times a week.

Age Management is very different. It is very patient-centered. There are diagnostic challenges to be sure, but they are the challenges of living better, not the challenges of diagnosing unusual cancers and rare infections. Shifting my focus from pathology to Age Management was a decision I couldn't make lightly.

I put a lot of thought into changing the direction of my practice. Part of my consideration was that I remembered when I was in medical school, several of my instructors were surprised by my choice of pathology as a specialty. They commented on what they saw as my excellent patient-oriented skills as a communicator, as an educator, and also as a problem solver. They said my diagnostic skills were excellent, but they said to me, "Why are you going to work in the laboratory? You should be with patients."

However, at the time, many years earlier, pathology was what appealed to me. I think it was that very problem-solving aspect my mentors mentioned that attracted me. I was very into the diagnostics. The tougher the problem the better. Only the most difficult diagnostic challenges require the skills of the pathologist. I was only a few years removed from my undergraduate experiences in my Cell Biology and Physiology major where I had become fascinated with the invisible world made real by the microscope. The way I looked at it then, I was with patients – just a little bit of them at a time.

But now, part of my own aging process had awakened an old interest in me. The desire for patient contact was revived, and I set off on a new course for myself, and one that would be an example for many of my patients.

Age Management Process

The ultimate goal of the Age Management Process is, of course, longevity. But longevity alone is not sufficient. No one wants to live to a ripe old age with discomfort and disability. Frail, fragile, and dependent is not how we imagine our retirement years. Rather, we want to waltz into old age with a song on our lips. We imagine ourselves striding into the room with a smile on our face and a spring in our step. We want to be the first on the dance floor and the last off the golf course. We see travel, enrichment, love – and lust – in our future; not wheel chairs, hearing aids, and diapers. Quality of life matters as much as quantity.

So if a doctor tells you that he has a supplement made from an ancient Chinese herb that will lengthen your telomeres allowing you to live to be 122 years old, this may at first be exciting, and, you think, worth the price. But if after some period of time you're getting older but not feeling better, you're going to have second thoughts about the side-effects, and the expense. Purchasing the newest and bestest super food with the highest ORAC value ever recorded may be exciting initially but when exactly does one feel better? [ORAC, the Oxygen Radical Absorbance Capacity, is a measure of how well it protects you from harmful chemical reactions] How will you know when it has worked? And if mice live longer when deprived of a full third of the calories necessary for a baseline metabolic rate, what's the likelihood that will work for humans who self regulate food intake? More on telomeres, super foods, and calorie restriction later. These concepts are alive more within the anti-aging camp rather than Age Management.

In AMM, our goal is to promote longevity while at the same time addressing current symptoms of aging. The symptoms of aging reflect underlying metabolic and hormonal changes such that the two - longevity and alleviating symptoms - are not mutually exclusive. Correcting the underlying hormonal and metabolic changes both improves symptom conditions and promotes longevity.

What You Can Do

Getting Started

I want to make it clear that the first step in any Age Management program is the individual's motivation. A motivated middle-aged or older person who is beginning to feel the symptoms of aging – and then decides that he is not willing to accept those symptoms – needs to find a doctor willing to work with him; someone who will take his concerns seriously. Essentially, he needs a specialist in age management because his regular doctor is not likely to be on top of the major developments that have come about in this new field in just over the last two decades.

What will send him looking for such a physician? What symptoms are most likely to move him to find solutions to his ailments and his slowing down? Read on.

Energy Level

Among the most important steps in age management medicine is to gather as much objective data as possible on the patient's current condition. But probably the most frequent concerns that patients come to me with are also the most subjective. In such instances though, no objective diagnostic test is available. I'm speaking of energy levesl.

Energy levels are entirely personal. They are based on experience and perception, and they are entirely individual and relative. So it becomes very important for the doctor to investigate with the patient exactly what low or lack of energy means to him, and how is that change in the patient's energy level affecting his life. It's essential to be specific about this information, and to get a complete and detailed description in the patient's own words. This is necessary in order to have something to evaluate, and to track over time. I reiterate that the physician needs to drill down through the patient's description of his declining energy, to ask questions the patient probably hasn't considered, to most closely define the facts, and the perceptions.

For those who have not yet had the good fortune to retire and who are still working, the most common manifestation of low energy level is a diminished ability to maintain their expected levels of functioning at work in the late afternoon. Someone who used to work efficiently and effectively until 6:00 in the evening may now be dragging by mid-afternoon. There can be actual fatigue, as in the desire to take a nap, and for others it can be that they notice that it is difficult to concentrate. Some people described this as being "in a fog." Still others simply find themselves daydreaming. For many people, there is a concomitant fear that they are experiencing intellectual impairment or a memory disorder.

For those working on commission – and especially the

self-employed – this perceived reduction in their effectiveness for a significant part of their day can mean serious adverse consequences for their income. For those with business partners, it can affect the quality of that relationship. For employees, it can cause problems with their employer, and even jeopardize their jobs. At the least, their perceived slacking off in the afternoons can result in sub-optimal employee evaluations, which could be the first steps down a long unhappy road.

At home, low-energy can affect our relationships with our spouse, our children, and grandchildren. Many of my patients tell me of complaints from their spouse about seeming remote, uninvolved, aloof or uncaring. (A related problem in this regard is also mood changes that often occur with aging; these will be discussed below.) Some patients recognize the changes in themselves but others are only aware of it via input from their family, friends, and colleagues.

More commonly though, it's the patients themselves who notice that, while they may have the desire to be more involved in their children's lives and activities, they just can't seem to find the energy that they used to have. Coaching the softball or soccer team. Going to karate class, music lessons, or art classes with their child. Traveling together to tournaments, camps, or events.

Then there are the grandparental relationships. The patients report that they can't seem to muster the energy to have their grand-kids over for a dinner, let alone for a weekend the way they used to do so easily.

Personal hobbies, sports, and social activities, also can suffer from a loss of energy. In my own case, in my thirties I would typically work until approximately six if I wasn't on call, and then routinely I would go to the gym for a workout or I would go for a run. Sometimes I had softball practice or a game after work. Then I would go home to make dinner and following that, I would practice the guitar until time for bed. By my late forties and early fifties though, I wasn't playing my guitar at all, I was no longer on a softball team, and I struggled to find the energy to run or go to the gym; except on weekends and days off. I just couldn't seem to muster the energy to work and workout on the same day. The fun that I experienced playing softball games in the past just wasn't enough to motivate me to get off the couch. Life wasn't quite as rich as it used to be. I felt like I was slowing down...and breaking down.

Intimacy and Sex Drive

Related to the above discussion but also a problem unto itself is decreased sexual energy. The desire for intimate relations with one's spouse or significant other also tends to decline with age. Loss of desire leads to a decreased frequency of sexual contact, and the proportion of couples living in a sexless relationship increases over time.

Needless to say, this loss of desire and intimacy can lead to diminished satisfaction with a relationship itself, and with life in general. Sex is a difficult issue to discuss for many in our culture. Most people would rather not talk about it than confront what they see as problems or inadequacies in their sex life. Many patients won't bring it up on their own, but I've seen genuine relief when I as their doctor opened the dialog and gave them a safe environment to discuss it.

Sexual Dysfunction

Libido aside, even when both partners have the desire and energy, sexual function declines over time. Probably the most frequent manifestations of sexual dysfunction in older women – other than loss of libido – are diminished vaginal lubrication, pain, itching, burning or general non-specific discomfort with intercourse. The discomfort symptoms are often secondary to the decreased lubrication but atrophy of the lining of the labia and vagina also contributes.

Though local symptoms are perhaps most common among women, a decline in the quality of the sexual experience is not an infrequent complaint. Less enjoyment of the experience overall – and specifically an inability to achieve orgasm in women who previously did not experience difficulty – are common issues among our aging population.

In men sexual problems manifest largely as erectile dysfunction. For some men, this is secondary to an underlying disease process such as peripheral vascular disease, diabetes, and/or hypertension. It is also often a symptom of a common psychological disorder, most frequently depression. This should be repeated: erectile dysfunction can be the result of such epidemic social conditions as stress and depression.

That said, erectile dysfunction can be an issue for many men who are not suffering from any of the above. Whatever the cause, the condition can be a source of considerable disappointment, frustration, and emotional distress, and for both partners.

Erectile dysfunction is typically defined medically as an inability to achieve or maintain an erection sufficient to make vaginal penetration. But there are many men who do not meet this specific definition but who nonetheless find that they are unable to obtain or maintain as firm an erection as they did when they were younger. They can achieve penetration to some degree on some occasions, but not as easily or as well as when they were younger.

As noted above, sex and ideas about sex are very important in our culture, and achieving an erection is viewed by most men as a basic human function. Any difficulty in performing what they once considered normal functions can be a source of serious frustration, on many levels. (You might remember in the movie M*A*S*H when the *swordsman* dentist (John Shuck) failed to perform and decided that he'd rather commit suicide than go on living *that way*.)

Contrary to popular belief, the inability to achieve orgasm also affects some men. It is not as frequent a complaint among men as women but it does occur. Either the problem had developed so slowly they didn't recognize it or they attributed it to some other psychological or relationship ailment. Some men are pleasantly shocked by the quality and quantity of their orgasms after starting testosterone therapy.

Over-Fat

Also a frequent first concern of people "feeling their age" is body composition, and by this I mean increasing body fat/weight and decreasing muscle mass/strength. I encounter concerns about fat much more often than about muscle condition. How many times have you heard one of your friends – or even yourself for that matter – complaining that as we get older it's so much easier to put on weight and so much more difficult to take it off? This is in fact a very real phenomenon related to physiologic and hormonal changes of aging that we will discuss below. The fact is that we aren't truly "overweight." Rather, we are over-fat. We don't have too much muscle or bone. We have too much fat. So I say, we aren't over-boned or over-muscled, we are over-fat.

Increased body fat is not just an issue of sitting on the couch for too many hours at the expense of exercise, or eating the wrong foods and too much of them. Extra body fat is a well-known risk factor for development of arterial diseases that lead to stroke, heart attack, kidney failure, and erectile dysfunction. Obesity, particularly visceral obesity – belly fat – leads to chronic inflammation and oxidative stress conditions that are a breeding ground for diseases such as diabetes, heart disease, hypertension, and cardio-vascular disease (CVD). (For more on oxidative stress, please go to page 83.)

Obesity is also a risk factor for the development of arthritis. In addition, in men obesity can lead to peripheral conversion of testosterone to estrogen, the female hormone. This means the possible feminization of the male body with characteristics such as breast development, but it more often counteracts the beneficial effects of the male hormone, testosterone.

And obesity is not just a physical problem. It can be greatly destructive to a person's confidence or self-image. Self-confidence and image issues are particularly important for those who work directly with the public, for example in a retail sales capacity, and also for those who are still searching for a mate.

The issue of muscle mass and strength is less often a primary concern but certainly can be for those like myself who have been physically active or athletic for their entire lives and wish to remain so. When they age, physically fit and active folks often feel that it takes much more effort to accomplish the same goals as twenty or thirty years ago. And they are right. Often they cannot accomplish the same goals at all. The required increase in effort and concomitant diminishing results lead to decreased motivation for exercise which combined with the diminished overall level of energy, in turn leads to more muscle mass loss, more fat gain and poorer self-image. As you can see, it can become a vicious downward cycle.

Muscle mass is important not only for aesthetics and athletic performance. Muscle also burns more calories when the body is at rest than any other tissue, and thus having more muscle mass helps prevent fat gain even when not exercising. Loss of muscle mass is the single biggest determinant of the decline in the at-rest metabolic rate that occurs with aging. And the decline in the metabolic rate contributes directly to fat gain.

In addition, as we age, loss of muscle, or sarcopenia, contributes to decreased strength and balance, both of which increase the probability of falls. Falls, of course, can lead to neurologic injuries such as subdural hematomas as well as to orthopedic injuries like a fractured hip. Such conditions and others are likely to lead to loss of independence, which is a huge fear among people getting older. Simply by virtue of rendering the activities of daily living more difficult, the weakness, frailty and loss of mobility of sarcopenia are significant even without an injury.

Mood

Mood changes, moodiness, or emotional lability – a sudden uncontrollable emotional swing - are common signs of aging. In women, this is strongly correlated with menopause. Its onset is over a relatively brief period of time; it's usually several months though it can stretch to a few years. In most cases, the onset and manifestations of menopause are obvious. Spouses often note frequent and wide mood swings that seem to have no correlation to the circumstances of the moment when they erupt. This makes it particularly difficult for the husband, who doesn't know where the change in mood comes from, or how to respond to it.

Anger and sadness are prominent emotions during these times. Outright depression is not infrequent.

Men experience mood changes as well – some call it the male version of menopause – but the onset is much more insidious, occurring over a number of years as opposed to a number of months. Men are more often described as irritable and moody but some of the words their wives (and friends and colleagues) use to describe them are withdrawn, unloving, sarcastic and argu-mentative. Like women, actual depression is sometimes a symptom of the aging man. Let's just say that the stereotype of the "grumpy old man" has at least some basis in reality.

Mood changes can affect not only marital relationships but also relationships with co-workers, friends, children, and other family members. But unlike the other symptoms of aging discussed above, patients often have little or no insight into the mood changes, and frequently are quite reticent to discuss the possibility that this is even an issue for them.

Sleep

Sleep quality declines with age. Subjectively, older adults report taking longer to fall asleep, waking up earlier, more time spent in bed, waking up in the middle of the night more often, taking naps, and decreased total sleep compared to younger adults. Using scientific measurement tools, research studies have found objective evidence that supports the subjective experiences described by older adults.

Sleep consists of two main phases: rapid eye movement (REM) sleep, and non-REM sleep. Non-REM sleep is divided into three progressively "deeper" stages: N1, N2, and N3. (Previous categorizations of sleep defined four levels, the last two of which have now been combined into N3). Typically, we cycle through each stage several times each night. Studies comparing sleep in older to younger adults found that older adults spend less time in deeper N3 stages of sleep, which is also referred to as slow-wave sleep (SWS).

The longest periods of SWS take place in the early parts of the night and are seen in greatest quantity in children and young adults. Younger adults deprived of SWS report feeling less refreshed. Studies also show that after a period of deprivation, for the next few undisturbed sleep cycles subjects experience a sharp rebound increase in SWS.

Slow-Wave Sleep diminishes with age and many older persons experience no SWS at all during their nightly sleep cycles.

Stress and Anxiety

On average, most Americans and Western Europeans acquire more sources of stress with age. It is easier to be worry free at twenty-five than at fifty-five. The young are more likely to be resilient because they aren't married, they are typically in entry-level positions at work, and they are more mobile in their attitudes. So a twenty-five-year-old who loses his job may find it less stressful because he is less likely to have a mortgage, a spouse, or children, whereas someone at fifty-five will have all of those "complications" and more...and less time to recover from such a reversal. Just ask an out-of-work fifty-five-year-old about his prospects for finding a new position, particularly in today's economy.

These are, of course, broad generalizations, but the larger issue is how much stress is generated for the individual experiencing the set-back, and how he subjectively experiences the stress. Older people may have a mature attitude toward dealing with such problems, but they also have aging factors that can make coping a more difficult task. One of those factors is that by living longer, someone is almost inevitably going to accumulate more stressors over the years. We know that the perception and the experience of stress do seem to change with age.

Stress research has shown that individuals who report the highest levels of perceived stress at initial evaluation also report the poorest physical health when reevaluated four years later. Additionally, this group is found to engage in the least amount of physical activity. It isn't clear if the stress leads to reduced activity which is what results in poor health or vice versa. But the current prevailing thought is that physical activity is an effective treatment for stress, and that relieving stress improves overall health.

Fatigue and perceived stress are also strongly correlated, but it isn't always clear how. Which comes first? Which is the result of the other? What is known is that these answers can vary with the individual. It is clear, that both stress and fatigue are vital factors in a person's overall health status.

There is an endocrine response to stress beginning in the brain and resulting in the release of cortisol (also known as cortisone) from the adrenal glands. The cortisol response mobilizes amino acids from protein stored in muscle, blood sugar (glucose) stored in the liver, and fatty acids from fat. The amino acids then enter the bloodstream for use as an immediate energy source. This stress response also helps the body to maintain blood pressure and limit excessive inflammation. During immediate or short term stress, this is an effective adaptive response. We encounter stress and the body mobilizes to meet the challenge. When the stressor is dealt with, cortisol levels and metabolic and immune processes return to normal.

But in our modern world, everyday demands of employment, financial issues, relationships, child care, dealing with aging parents, low sleep, and empty calories can produce cortisol levels that are chronically elevated, and serious negative health effects ensue. There is very good scientific and medical evidence to show that chronically-elevated cortisol levels are associated with:

Obesity

High blood pressure

Diabetes

Fatigue

Depression

Moodiness

Irregular menstrual periods in pre-menopausal women

Diminished libido

Cognitive decline

Dealing effectively with stress is among the main goals of an Age Management regimen. The best therapy, of course, is to remove stressors. But it may not be possible to "remove" your mother-in-law or to leave your job, so a person has to find a way to deal with the stress. Non-pharmacologic approaches are best because the drugs that are most often prescribed – anxiolytics and psychotropics – do nothing to the cortisol stress response, and can lead to dependence. Different individuals respond to different approaches, but I have seen good results with hypnotherapy, meditation, and yoga...all without harmful side effects.

Dementia/Alzheimer's

It is widely, but not universally, accepted that declines in memory and cognitive abilities are a normal consequence of aging. It appears to be true across cultures and other mammalian species. Some older adults appear to have difficulties greater than others but not so pronounced as to meet the definition of Alzheimer's disease. Various terms have been proposed to describe such instances including mild cognitive impairment, late-life forgetfulness and possible dementia, among others. To make the distinction then, let's take a quick look at what is dementia and Alzheimer's.

Dementia is a more general term than Alzheimer's. The simplest definition of dementia is loss of short term memory but retained long term memory. We've all met the "old codger" who can tell you precisely, in exquisite detail, again and again, what he had for lunch the day of his high school graduation, but he doesn't recall that he just related the story two minutes ago. People with more advanced dementia may have difficulty with even more basic thinking processes. They may not be able to think well enough, for example, to perform normal activities of daily living that were never previously a problem. Problem-solving ability may suffer. Personality may change, often manifesting as an inability to control emotions, perhaps with the person becoming easily agitated. They may show poor judgment or have difficulty with visual spatial orientation, e.g. lose the ability to read a clock or, worse yet, recognize a face.

Dementia can result from a variety of brain insults including vascular disease resulting in multiple small strokes, brain injuries, metabolic disorders secondary to lung, liver or kidney dysfunction, or degenerative diseases. Most frequent among all, though, is Alzheimer's. But what specifically constitutes it is difficult to define.

There is no single diagnostic test available for though Alzheimer's. The specific medical diagnosis can only be established at autopsy. There is no blood test or brain imaging procedure that can establish a diagnosis of Alzheimer's. In the absence of a diagnostic test, doctor's criteria involve an assessment that (1) the onset is slow over a long period, (2) is clearly progressive, and (3) the symptoms involve more than one of the following:

Short term memory impairment;

Difficulty finding words when speaking;

Visual spatial impairment;

Executive thinking impairment.

Executive functions are things like the ability to analyze a task, plan how to accomplish it, organize as needed to get it done, adjust the plan if necessary, and complete the task.

Mild cognitive impairment (MCI) is an intermediate stage between the "expected" cognitive decline of normal aging and the more pronounced decline of dementia. It involves problems with memory, language, thinking, and judgment. Processing speed, reasoning, memory, and executive functions are most affected.

Symptoms of MCI can include:

Difficulty performing more than one task at a time;

Difficulty solving complex problems or making decisions;

Forgetting recent events or conversations;

Taking longer to perform more difficult mental activities.

As you can see, there is considerable overlap between what is considered "normal" brain aging, MCI, and Alzheimer's. As you will also note, the criteria are highly subjective. Obvious Alzheimer's is easy to spot. Non-professionals can easily diagnose it with a minimum understanding of the symptoms. It is the more subtle forms of cognitive impairment that are difficult to spot and diagnose with certainty. But, importantly, it is the early cases that respond best to intervention.

Given all the above, my philosophy is to regard all age-related cognitive impairment as abnormal. In those with none, my goal is prevention. In those with early or minimal changes, my goal is improvement or at least to limit progression. The sad truth is that once someone has clear-cut dementia, little can be done.

Chronic Inflammation

Inflammation isn't an aging "symptom" per se but it is an adverse condition that comes with aging nonetheless. Localized inflammation as seen in the lungs in pneumonia, joints in arthritis, and in the skin with an abscess are patently obvious problems that arise as people age. Pneumonia manifests as coughing and shortness of breath, arthritis with pain and limitation of range of motion, and an abscess causes pain, redness and draining pus.

Sometimes the site of inflammation is less obvious but the patient may have systemic signs such as fever, shaking chills, or drenching sweats. Laboratory tests for inflammation - white blood cell count (WBC), erythrocyte sedimentation rate (ESR), and C-reactive protein (CRP) - show elevated numbers. The high-sensitivity CRP is the preferred screening test in healthy adults.

But what of the person with an elevated lab test value but no clinical signs or symptoms of a localized source nor any systemic symptoms? Until little less than ten years ago, that situation was a conundrum. But follow-up studies have shown that these individuals are at higher risk for arterial diseases of all sorts, even if they are entirely asymptomatic at the time of the initial evaluation.

The process of inflammation is now believed to be the causative process that precedes the development of atherosclerosis. That is, the inflammation, even if it doesn't produce obvious symptoms, can be doing deadly work out of sight of normal preliminary tests. This process begins with an injury or change in the innermost layer of the artery wall, called the intima, which is lined by a layer of cells called endothelial cells. Inflammation causes an alteration in the intimal layer that increases adhesion of WBCs, oxidized LDL (low-density lipoprotein or "bad cholesterol"), and platelets to the endothelium.

In layman's terms, cholesterol does not deposit in a normal artery wall. The artery has to be damaged first.

Possible antecedents to this process include: free radical damage; high blood pressure and its pro-inflammatory effects; and advanced glycation end-products (AGEs), the result of an oxidative reaction with glucose.

Atherosclerosis – what happens when the artery walls thicken, harden and narrow on the inside with cholesterol – is the underlying process behind heart attacks, strokes, peripheral vascular disease, kidney failure, some types of dementia, and erectile dysfunction. Inflammation may also play a role in osteopenia/osteoporosis, insulin resistance, frailty/physical disability, cognitive decline, and overall mortality.

What can cause modest elevations of inflammation that are seen with aging? Many of the cases, though by no means all, include belly fat, lower sex steroid hormones, smoking, periodontal disease, sedentary lifestyle, low omega-3/high-saturated fat diet, depression, and anxiety.

Aches, Pains, and Stiffness

Like low energy, these discomfort concerns are both frequent and subjective. And like energy, they are typically multi-factorial. Sure, there are some cases of arthritis in the group. But it's the generalized sense of feeling "stiff as a board" or "frozen up" or "sore all over" that I refer to here.

Objectively, an AMM physician has a few things to rule

out in this regard like Parkinson's disease when stiffness is prominent, or rheumatoid arthritis and systemic lupus when pain is greatest. Those aside, we examine for range of motion limitations, pain, and tenderness that can limit ability to exercise or worse yet, to conduct the activities that we consider part of daily living.

Let me tell you from personal experience – and I know many of you have had this yourselves – that at times I've had difficulty just getting up out of a chair and walking upright. It can be very frustrating. As a pathologist, I would frequently spend an hour or more at a time at my microscope. Afterward, when I rose from my chair, I would often be stooped over and unable to walk upright for several minutes. More than once a colleague passing me in the hallway would inquire if I was okay! I was about as limber as flag pole. This was a big motivator for me to take an interest in AMM. and I've had dramatic success at improving this previously troublesome part of my life.

For most folks like me, the problem is some combination of stress, chronic inflammation, low (but not necessarily deficient) growth hormone (GH), and insufficient commitment to a stretching routine. All can easily be successfully addressed. Physical therapists, massage therapists, and yoga instructors – in person or in videos – can be excellent sources for learning stretching routines specific to your unique needs.

Osteopenia/Osteoporosis

Like inflammation, loss of bone mass is not exactly a symptom in the sense that people don't feel it happening, and they are not typically aware of it until an obvious manifestation, like a bone fracture, occurs. It is more of a peril of aging than a symptom. Falls with fractures are a major cause of loss of mobility and independence with aging.

Bone mass is created throughout our youth until approximately age thirty, and after that there is a steady decline over time. With the exception of an accelerated loss that occurs in the peri-menopausal and early post-menopausal period, bone loss occurs equally in both men and women. We can maximize bone mass when young with appropriate exercise and nutrition, but typically most folks around thirty aren't paying much attention to their future health. But later, when we do begin to pay attention, appropriate diet and exercise can help slow the rate of bone loss. Fractures are not inevitable and can be avoided with more attention to future health issues when we are still young.

Nutritionally, both vitamin D and calcium are essential for building and maintaining bone mass. Adequate protein intake is also important.

Exercise is also key to prevention, but not just any exercise. Resistance training is the best. Even hand weights, leg weights, free weights, resistance bands, et cetera, are adequate if used often enough, and with adequate resistance.

But even with good nutrition and exercise, as we age, we are inevitably swimming upstream against the critical changes in important hormones such as GH, estrogen, testosterone, and DHEA, the sex steroid hormone dehydroepiandrosterone.

Basic Biology 101

It seems then that aging renders us tired, lazy, weak, fat, flabby, grumpy, and asexual, along with giving us bad arteries and weak bones. Not a pretty sight, I'd aver. Let's see how we get there. First, know that hormonal and metabolic changes are critical to the process. And to better understand, lets review a simplified bit of basic biology first. Don't be too concerned with the details, but I think a brief review will enhance your understanding of the aging process. And no, there won't be a test.

Cell Biology

Cells are the basic structural unit of life. They consume energy, produce waste, and can reproduce themselves. Individual organisms – from humans and other mammals to fish, amphibians, reptiles, birds and worms – are made up of organs such as brain, heart, lungs or gills, kidneys, et cetera. Organs are constructed of tissues which in turn are made up of cells.

Think of an individual person or animal as a city which has neighborhoods (organs) composed of homes (tissues) made up of rooms (cells). Cells have even smaller structures for energy production or manufacturing proteins, and a nucleus where the DNA and other reproductive material are housed.

DNA is nothing more than a blueprint. It's a set of plans for your cells. Every cell in your body has the same DNA. Every cell – from nerve cells to eye cells to stomach and bone cells – has exactly the same DNA. The same information. The same blueprint. Yet all those cells are remarkably and obviously different. That is because each cell type uses only that portion of the entire blueprint relevant to its own function. How each cell knows just what part of the blueprint to read is a fascinating topic but beyond the scope of this discussion.

As mentioned, DNA is housed in the nucleus of the cell. The DNA is a coiled molecule made up of two complementary chains of nucleic acid subunits. A series of these subunits linked together in a unique sequence constitutes a gene. One gene encodes the instructions for building one protein. Its like Morse code. The sequence of dots, dashes and spaces determines the message.

Chromosomes are the structures within the nucleus that house the DNA strands. One chromosome holds multiple genes, and there are multiple chromosomes per cell.

Proteins can be structural or functional. Functional proteins are the movers and shakers of the cellular world. They make stuff happen. Most are enzymes or hormones. An enzyme is a catalyst, an enabling substance that allows a biochemical reaction to occur under conditions that would not otherwise be permissive. Enzymes are essential for normal cellular activities.

A hormone is an intercellular chemical messenger, produced in one location, acting at another, and regulating cellular function. Organs and tissues in widely disparate locations communicate via both the nervous system and hormones. And hormones communicate with the nervous system creating an integrated, finely-tuned whole.

Structural proteins are building blocks for all sorts of cell structures including cell membranes as well as nuclear membranes, chromosomes and others.

Hormonic Convergence

Its just a bit of an oversimplification, but generally true nonetheless, that aging is accompanied by decreasing levels of "good" hormones with increasing levels of "bad" hormones.

The "bad" is principally insulin. I don't wish to slur insulin's good name because we would certainly have a hard time getting along without it. But we can get too much of a good thing. As much as I love the Beatles, sometimes I think I just can't handle hearing *Hey Jude* one more time!

The "good" hormones in this regard include estrogen and progesterone in women, testosterone in men, and DHEA, GH, melatonin and thyroid in both genders.

Growth Hormone

As its name implies, growth hormone (GH) plays a critical role in the physical growth of infants, children, and teenagers to adulthood. Each of us grows differently based on our genetics but when we are done, we're done. There is little growth role left for GH after we stop growing which for most of us, is by about the age of twenty, tops. After that, there is a precipitous drop off in the amount of GH that can be measured in the blood.

It turns out though, that lower levels of GH are maintained even after adolescence and on into adulthood. It doesn't entirely disappear. At that stage in life, GH is supporting the maintenance and healing of soft tissues including bone, muscle, ligament and tendon. (Yes, bone is a soft tissue when it is not mineralized. Bone is a living tissue with a connective tissue framework that becomes mineralized).

GH also has a substantial positive effect on mood. Maybe that is why it seems easier to feel less stressed and to be happier when younger. We know that throughout adulthood though, GH production slowly falls, and in older age can actually become deficient, resulting in the onset of aging symptoms.

GH deficiency manifests as decreased overall quality of life, fatigue, and alteration of body composition. Abnormalities may be pronounced. Sufferers may experience:

A higher level of body fat, especially belly fat

Changes in the makeup of the blood cholesterol: more bad and less good

Decreased sexual interest and function

Fatigue

Anxiety and depression

Less muscle mass

Less strength and exercise stamina

Reduced bone density

Sex Hormones

Sex hormones also decline with age. In women, estrogen and progesterone levels remain fairly stable from puberty through menopause. Then they fall precipitously during the peri-menopausal period and that fall is often accompanied by some combination of:

Hot flashes in almost all menopausal women

Night sweats

Wide, sudden and often unexpected mood swings

Anxiety and depression

Sleep disturbance

Decreased libido, sexual responsiveness and quality of the sexual experience

Vaginal dryness, burning, itching or pain

Weight gain

Increased risk of cardiovascular disease

Loss of bone mass

These changes occur over several months to a few years with a fairly easily identifiable onset around age fifty for most women. Any woman reading this who has been through it doesn't need me to tell her how debilitating these symptoms can be. Men can relate to most of them but not the hot flashes. And these can be particularly vexing to some women.

Men's sex hormone, testosterone, also falls with age but at a much more gradual rate. So much so that the onset of associated symptoms is gradual and less pronounced and can often go unnoticed for years. Testosterone levels peak around about age twenty for most men. Levels decline at about a half-percent per year during the twenties, then at about one percent per year thereafter. A man of fifty then has probably about 25% less testosterone production as he did at twenty.

In addition though, production of the binding protein to which testosterone is attached, Sex Hormone Binding Globulin or SHBG, increases with age. Bound testosterone lasts longer but the binding protein also inactivates it. A vast majority of the testosterone in the blood at any time is bound to SHBG. And it is only the unbound, or free, portion that is active.

So as a man ages, he experiences falling total testosterone with rising SHBG. The net result is a double whammy such that by age fifty, a man's active testosterone has fallen by half or more.

This is often referred to as hypogonadism or, less often, andropause. Symptoms include:

Decrease in muscle mass

Decreased sex drive

Erectile dysfunction

Fatigue

Difficulty concentrating

Development of breast tissue (gynecomastia)

Loss of bone mass (osteoporosis)

Difficulty concentrating

Though the predominant male sex hormone is testosterone, men also make small amounts of estrogen from their testosterone. The enzyme aromatase brings about the conversion.

Aromatase is in higher concentration in fatty tissues and this accounts for the propensity of obese men to have higher levels of female hormone and also sometimes to develop breast tissue. Estrogen effects counter those of testosterone and can contribute to lower libido.

DHEA

Dehydroepiandrosterone (DHEA) is a member of the sex steroid hormone family like estrogen and testosterone. DHEA is the hormone present in the greatest amount in blood. Levels peak at around age twenty, then decline by roughly 10% per decade. By age seventy, DHEA levels reach a relatively stable level of 10% to 20% of a young adult level. Think about that. An 80% to 90% reduction at seventy. That's pretty dramatic.

In the 1960s, DHEA was found to be an intermediate molecule in the pathway to testosterone production. This finding sparked much interest in DHEA supplementation as a bodybuilding or athletic performance enhancer, but its effectiveness was limited by the fact that it also may serve as an ingredient in making estrogen. High-dose supplementation seems to produce more estrogen than testosterone. These findings have led to a conventional wisdom in traditional medicine circles that DHEA is of no value in aging patients.

It turns out though, that DHEA has biologic effects all its own that are entirely unrelated to its role as a precursor molecule. This is worth discussing in just a bit of detail since recommending DHEA supplementation is somewhat controversial.

In women studied over time, initial DHEA levels are directly related to measures of well-being, cognitive function, and functional status at subsequent follow-ups two and again at four years later.

In men studied over time, DHEA levels are inversely related to total mortality risk and also risk of dying of cardiovascular disease. One study of men over fifty with no prior history of heart disease, found that the men with low DHEA were 3.3 times more likely to die of a cardiovascular event in the subsequent 12 years than men with a normal DHEA. So if the men with normal levels had a 10% risk let's say, then the men with low levels had a 33% risk.

Better news still for those inclined to supplement with DHEA is that in one research study, individuals with DHEA blood levels of approximately 70% or more above the low levels associated with risk, have an approximately one-third reduction in mortality from any cause, and a nearly 50% reduction in mortality from cardiovascular disease! Other studies have shown similar though somewhat less dramatic findings.

Most of the research with regard to mortality and vascular disease has been conducted in men. Where women have been included, the associations were not as strong for cardiovascular disease or mortality from all causes.

Because it is a member of the androgen family, DHEA has been examined as a possible erectile dysfunction (ED) treatment. Not all studies have shown a beneficial effect but supplementation with DHEA has been shown to improve ED problems in men with high blood pressure.

Some research studies have demonstrated a correlation between Alzheimer's Disease (AD) and DHEA levels. In patients with pre-existing AD, those with higher DHEA levels perform better in cognitive function testing. This is an exciting finding because it indicates the possibility of a cause and effect relationship. However, AD patients treated with DHEA have, to date, not shown improvement in cognitive function. At present then, I don't think it is fair to say that DHEA can be used to improve cognition with age, but there is some evidence indicating it may be preventative.

Low DHEA levels also correlate with lower bone mineral density (BMD) and osteoporosis risk. Some, but not all, DHEA supplementation studies have improved BMD in women and men with osteoporosis.

DHEA supplementation has been found safe even at relatively high doses.

Melatonin

Melatonin is a hormone synthesized in the pineal gland of the brain. Its synthesis and secretion have a pronounced circadian rhythm strongly correlated with the light-dark cycle. The normal nighttime secretion of melatonin, known to play an important role in the sleep-wake cycle, gradually decreases with age, resulting in reduced sleep efficiency and an increase in sleep disturbances with age.

There is also a consistent relationship between growth hormone secretion and slow-wave-sleep (SWS) quality. It has been shown that growth hormone levels diminish in conjunction with impaired slow-wave quality. Also, there is a correlation between retaining SWS quality and well-maintained blood growth hormone levels.

Thus, age-related sleep disturbance is significant; not only for its contribution to diminished quality of life, but also because it may contribute to adult-onset growth hormone deficiency. The perception of fatigue that follows poor sleep, combined with mood changes and low-energy, can represent a significant detriment to quality of life. It can also contribute to increased perception of anxiety and stress and no one needs more of that.

Thyroid Hormone

In adults, thyroid hormone helps regulate metabolic rate. Higher levels stimulate heart rate and calorie consumption. Lower levels result in the opposite. Symptoms of low thyroid hormone levels include:

Fatigue

Weakness

Weight gain

Depression

Irritability

Memory loss

Decreased libido

Thyroid hormones do not show the precipitous decline of the female sex hormones nor the steady decline of male sex hormones and melatonin. But the frequency of diseases resulting in low thyroid hormone production does increase with age.

Insulin

Insulin levels do not normally decline with age. To the contrary, in today's modern western culture of sedentary lifestyles with high-calorie, low-nutrient foods, insulin levels can climb in obese individuals, and are intimately involved in the genesis of adult onset or Type 2 diabetes (AODM). The cause of AODM is multi-factorial. Clearly, there is a genetic predisposition. Obesity and lack of physical activity are significant risk factors. But a critical first step is insulin resistance.

Insulin is released by the pancreas in response to rising blood sugar levels. Blood sugar rises normally after eating but it rises more so after high-calorie meals and meals rich in sugar. The pancreas responds with higher insulin levels following high-calorie or sugary meals.

Insulin is extremely effective at driving blood sugar levels down. It circulates in the blood, interacting with the insulin-sensitive tissues in the body, liver, muscle, and fat. These cells recognize insulin and interact with it. Its important to understand that the main message of insulin is "store and save." Not just bringing down blood sugar, but storing energy as fat and saving fat already stored are its principal goals. A muscle cell or a liver cell gets that message and makes carbohydrate stores. Fat cells respond by making...surprise, fat.

If frequent high-calorie, sugary meals are consumed, more and more insulin is released until all insulin responsive cells approach saturation. Over time, when exposed to frequent insulin surges, cells also "down regulate" or decrease their ability to respond to insulin. The net result of down regulation and saturation is insulin resistance. Blood sugar rises despite the fact the pancreas can still make insulin. Its just that the cells are no longer able to respond. This is the first step on the path to adult diabetes and it all begins with too many empty calories.

Insulin and Diet

Given the significance of elevated insulin and resistance to it, it would be useful to have a way to quantify the insulin response to various foods so as to avoid eating too much of the ones that create an exaggerated response. And in fact we have a way to measure how much a particular food drives up blood sugar levels; it is the glycemic index (GI). It is the ratio of the rise of blood sugar of a particular food compared to a reference point; typically blood sugar itself, or glucose.

Glucose is arbitrarily assigned a value of 100 and other foods are measured against it. Carbohydrates that break down quickly during digestion and release blood sugars (glucose) rapidly into the bloodstream have a high GI. Carbohydrates that break down more slowly, releasing glucose more gradually into the bloodstream, have a low GI.

Glycemic load (GL) is a measure of the total amount of carbohydrate consumed in a serving or meal.

We Are What We Eat

Humans have been around in our current form for

approximately three million years. Throughout most of that history we have been hunter-gatherers, eating lean meats we could procure by hunting, and also fruits, nuts, and vegetables we foraged from the ground or in low-hanging trees. We didn't settle down and begin growing grains until about ten thousand years ago. For the majority of our evolutionary history, we were not eating grains to any significant extent.

Human bodies are expert at processing lean meat and fruits and vegetables, all of which are low-glycemic foods. Evolutionarily speaking, we are not well suited to processing grains which are typically higher glycemic index foods.

This is where you can really take responsibility for the fuel you take into your body. You don't have to be dogmatic about it, but at least be aware. Pay attention to what you eat and how much of each substance.

Here are some everyday foods and their glycemic index:

White rice	93
Brown rice	87
Corn cold breakfast cereals	72-92
Oatmeal from rolled oats	up to 75
Potatoes	high 80s to 100+

Compare those numbers to broccoli/lettuce, cabbage,

mushrooms/onions/bell peppers which are rated at 10.

Or chickpeas/ kidney beans/lentils which are under 30.

Meats and fishes have a GI of zero.

Additional examples of high-GI foods include sugars, syrups, honey, soft drinks, muffins, pancakes, waffles, croissants, white bread, bagels, graham crackers, cupcakes, doughnuts, croissants, potatoes, macaroni and cheese, pizza, popcorn, cakes, pies, cookies, pretzels, and ice cream. Note the high proportion of baked goods and cereals; they are all made with grains.

Cattle are an excellent example of the effects of grain on fat deposition. Commercially-raised cattle spend the vast majority of their lives grazing openly on grass and any other green stuff they lay their eyes on. Then for about the last month before slaughter, they are brought into pens and fed corn and grains - high glycemic index foods. It is during this brief period at the end of their lives that they pack on a majority of their fat that we try so hard to avoid.

On the LiveBetterLonger.info website, I have posted an image that graphically displays the effects of large quantities of dietary grain in a side-by-side comparison. This is the difference that approximately three to four weeks of high GI diet makes to cattle. Imagine what it does to humans for years and years and years.

Confusion over What to Eat

Since the discovery of a relationship between dietary fat and cholesterol with blood cholesterol and fat levels – and also the recognition that these are correlated with risk for heart attack and stroke – the #1 public health dietary message has been that to avoid fats, and meats have been targeted as a source. There has been an emphasis on increasing consumption of fruits, vegetables and grains. This has inadvertently led, I believe, to an increased consumption of simple carbohydrates that contribute, to some degree at least, to the obesity and diabetes epidemics.

To avoid dietary fat, many folks have eschewed eggs and meat for breakfast in favor of cold cereal, oatmeal, bagels or croissants. Some just have a doughnut or pastry. For lunch or dinner they have pasta - i.e., white flour - or potatoes and rice, which are all high GI foods, and we have seen how such foods stimulate fat storage. The public health message to consume a low-fat diet has led us to a turn away from meats and toward high carbohydrate items, especially grains. To whatever extent we have followed that advice it has contributed to increased obesity and all its consequences, e.g. diabetes, heart disease, stroke, and kidney failure.

Primary Cause of Aging

We've seen that there are physiologic changes in hormonal status and metabolism that lead to the symptoms of aging. But what is the underlying mechanism? Why does this happen? The reality is that we still have no definitive explanation for the aging process or its underlying mechanisms. Though none is known with any degree of certainty, there are several theories, largely based on animal models, population studies, and evaluations of humans demonstrating marked longevity. They are worth reviewing here since some have recently received much public attention but not too much scrutiny.

It is easy to imagine the obvious practical, ethical, and economic obstacles to the long term follow-up studies that would be required to investigate the determinants of the human life span. Physiologically and health-wise, humans peak at between about twenty and thirty years of age. (Thank goodness, the same cannot necessarily be said about our decision-making and judgment!) Yet our average expected life span now approaches eighty or more. It is difficult to see how it would be practical or ethical to intrude on people with tests for fifty to sixty years of follow-up to acquire the necessary data.

For that matter, how does one ethically justify supplying a possibly life-extending intervention to one test group but not another for fifty years in order to make a rational comparison? And how would it be possible to control all the variables influencing survival that could affect free living humans?

Given these rather sizeable deterrents, most research

has been done instead on other organisms like yeast, the nematode worm, the fruit fly, and the mouse. But how applicable are such results to humans? We don't know. What we do know is that there is wide variability in how different organisms respond to environmental stimuli, and also to human-contrived interventions like medications.

The human studies that have been carried out have largely been retrospective. That is, beginning with long-lived individuals then looking back at their lives to see what they might have in common. The problem with this approach though, is the question of what variables should a researcher set about to examine? What if the most important ones are those that have not yet been discovered or even imagined? Important trends can easily be missed, and insignificant trends can be accorded undue importance.

The consensus view, not uniformly adhered to as you will see, is that there is no single "cause" of aging. No unique factor or risk can be singled out. As with most living processes, the cause of aging appears to be multifactorial. Chief among the factors is genetics.

Genetics

Observations of geographically-distinct populations such as on the island of Okinawa and in the Caucasus

Mountains region – areas where longevity is greater than the world norm – have indicated a genetic basis for longevity. Rural and geographically isolated populations such as these are relatively ethnically homogeneous. The fact that separate, geographically-isolated, ethnically-homogeneous populations stand out for a particular trait is good presumptive evidence that that trait is genetically-based. This is especially true because the two regions are far distant from each other, the lifestyles and dietary habits vary substantially, and the genetic pools in each area are different. Okinawa is Far East Asia. The Caucasus region includes Armenia, Chechnya, Azerbaijan, Georgia and portions of Russia, Iran and Turkey among others. The people of the Caucasuses share more with the European peoples, and those of the Middle East than with those of the Far East. Though they share a longevity trait, each is a distinct population.

There is already considerable research that has revealed that the genes you are born with are likely among the most significant determinants of how long you *might* live, but not necessarily how long you *will* live. We inherit an opportunity, not a guarantee. Studies of twins and long-lived sibling sets suggest that the average set of genetic variations enables the average human to live on average well into his eighties. Those with the good fortune to inherit a better than average set of genetic variations can certainly live to 100. Studies also show that people who take full advantage of their average gene set – that is, by living a healthy lifestyle – are going to spend the majority of those years in good health.

Of course, we also know that all too many people will not press their natural advantage but instead will counteract their genetic gifts with poor eating habits and a lack of exercise, and the results point to a notably lower average life expectancy and relatively more time spent in poor health. It's all about personal responsibility – being informed and following good habits.

Genetic variations probably operate in two distinct ways: an absence of factors that predispose to disease, and secondly, possessing variations that confer disease resistance.

Other studies on centenarians have revealed that extraordinary longevity is strongly associated with having a young mother! Being born to a mother twenty-five or younger at the time of birth is the strongest predictor of living a long life. Even among folks who have reached the age of seventy-five, the likelihood of reaching a hundred is higher amongst those born to a woman younger than twenty-six. It is thought that this is related to egg quality, which has been shown to begin to decline as early as age thirty. This same relationship holds true as well with other animals. It's fascinating to me that an event so many years prior could have such profound, long-lasting consequences.

Body weight at age thirty is also a strong predictor of the likelihood of reaching the century mark in age.

Being in the top fifteen percentile of body weight at the age of thirty is a strong negative predictor of reaching one hundred. This may to some extent be genetic but clearly can also be substantially influenced by lifestyle so it is difficult to statistically tease out the significance of the genetic component.

As interesting as these observations may be, and as strongly indicative of a genetic basis for aging as they are, still none of this tells us the specific mechanisms we inherit or how specific processes are affected by our genes.

Metabolism

Genetics aside, enhanced resistance to oxidative stress (see below) and increased xenobiotic metabolism are recurring, but not exclusive, findings among different long-lived species.

Xenobiotic metabolism is the set of metabolic pathways that modify the chemical structure of foreign and possibly toxic materials we encounter, e.g., drugs and poisons. These reactions are how our body acts to detoxify potentially harmful foreign substances by chemically transforming them. Animal experiments and observations have found that those best able to detoxify harmful substances have a longevity advantage.

Typically, talk of "toxins" conjures up images of crop dusters spraying fields or chemical plants spewing forth clouds of volatile fume. But humans evolved such detoxifying processes long before man-made toxins and poisons ever existed. The advantage must arise from an ability to process naturally-occurring substances.

Over the millennia, plants and fungi have developed thousands of natural compounds that protect them from enemies. A plant's natural toxins are intended to guard against threats from predators or disease, e.g. insects and fungi. An example of a natural toxin is a poison called aflatoxin. It is produced by a mold that grows on grains and nuts. It is a potent liver toxin and gram for gram, among the most potent carcinogens known. The FDA has set a maximum permissible level for aflatoxin requiring American food manufacturers to have quality control processes in place to prevent or minimize contamination. The point being that the human ability to process foreign substances has evolved over millions of years, and is not related at all to the post-industrialized world, but rather is a response to the defense mechanisms of human food sources. So humans were able to survive eating plants that just made us sick instead of killing us

Oxidative Stress

If you're like me, you probably recall the local fire captain coming to your elementary school and giving the fire safety talk. It seems to me that he always mentioned the fire triangle: fuel, oxygen and an ignition source. A fire consumes fuel to produce heat and carbon dioxide.

In like manner, we humans produce our energy by combining fuel with oxygen and producing heat and CO_2. We acquire fuel via food intake, oxygen from the air in our lungs. But what is our ignition? It's the spark of life that we all were given when we were conceived and which is passed along from generation to generation like the Olympic torch. It may have begun with divine intent or it may have been a lightning strike in a primordial soup of macromolecules and minerals. But in any event we all have it.

Our bodies are not at room temperature. We normally exist above room temperature at 98.6 degrees Fahrenheit because we're constantly producing heat by consuming our fuel. This chemical reaction has been ongoing since the first human and has been passed along via reproduction ever since. And that reaction produces byproducts called reactive oxygen species (ROS) and these include free radicals.

I think just about anyone with a passing interest in health and nutrition has heard of antioxidants. Well, the ROS mentioned above are the "oxidants" we need to protect ourselves from with antioxidants. ROS are highly-chemically reactive molecules containing oxygen. As noted, ROS form as a natural byproduct of metabolism. But they can also occur as a consequence of multiple different adverse events including trauma, infections, inflammation, and exposure to environmental agents. "Oxidative stress" refers to the negative effects of ROS on biologic structures and processes.

If ROS are not somehow inactivated, their high chemical reactivity can damage lipids (oils and fats), proteins, carbohydrates and DNA. Due to their high content of both lipids and proteins, cellular membranes are especially vulnerable. ROS can also interact with DNA and cause several types of damage, possibly resulting in mutations or ineffective cell division and cell death.

The sum total of such chemical reactions is called oxidative stress. Most cells can tolerate a mild degree of oxidative stress, because they have sufficient antioxidant defense capacity and repair systems that recognize and remove oxidized molecules. Oxidative stress damage by ROS is counteracted by our own antioxidants, and by nutritional antioxidants from diet. Oxidants and antioxidants normally exist in balance, but if the scales tilt toward the oxidants, molecular damage, cellular dysfunction, and disease may follow.

What has received perhaps the most popular attention in the antioxidant story is the possible role of free radicals in the development of coronary artery disease and strokes. Free radicals and coronary artery disease both can develop from atherosclerosis. And the development of atherosclerosis requires not just cholesterol in any form, but specifically, oxidized LDL (low-density lipoprotein or "bad cholesterol").

Although our bodies make many of their own en-dogenous antioxidants, there are numerous nutritional sources as well, most notably fruits and vegetables, and whole grains to a lesser extent. Population studies have revealed that societies where fruits and vegetable comprise a high proportion of total food bulk have lower rates of cancer and heart disease than the modern American and western European.

Such observations have led many scientific inves-tigators to believe that oxidative stress may play a sig-nificant, if not predominant, role in the aging process.

Telomeres

A recently-published, widely-read book on aging claimed to have found the ultimate cause of aging: short telomeres. Not only does the book report the cause, but also its cure, which it says is the herb astragulus. Given the success of the book and the growing acceptance within the anti-aging community of the primacy of short telomeres in the aging process, this is worth discussing at some length.

Telomeres are chromosomal structures that play a crit-ical role in cell reproduction. They are the attachment point for the enzyme that duplicates DNA before a cell divides and with each division, a small portion of the telomere is lost.

It has also been observed that short telomeres are seen

in aged cells and longer ones in younger cells. Given these observations, many have theorized that telomere shortening plays a role in cellular aging, and therefore, presumably in the aging of the entire organism.

We lose most of our telomere length, though, before we are born. Stem cells have very long telomeres but they become markedly foreshortened during the rapid growth that occurs with gestation. So we are born with a majority of telomere length already lost.

Interestingly, in the early 1960s, it was noted by Dr. Leonard Hayflick at Stanford University that cells grown in culture make only a limited number of cell divisions before they die. There appeared to be a maximum number of cell divisions a cell could make before becoming senescent and dying. This was dubbed the Hayflick limit and it seemed to dovetail nicely with the correlation of short telomeres with cell death. It seemed the Hayflick limit was reached when telomeres reached a critically short length.

Also of note, malignant cells typically have longer telomeres than their benign counterparts. Malignant cells also live longer in tissue culture than benign cells, usually indefinitely. The current thinking is that long telomeres *allow*, but do not necessarily *cause*, malignant transformation.

In a fully-mature individual, cells divide presumably either to balance normal cell loss or in response to injury. But different tissues turn over at different rates.

Blood forming cells and those that line our intestinal tracts do so at much higher rates than most others. With rare exception, central nervous system neurons seem never to turn over at all.

Combining this genetic knowledge with the observations of Dr. Hayflick, molecular geneticists proposed the theory that the loss of telomeres and the subsequent inability of cells to reproduce, are the ultimate causes of cell death and that cell death is the ultimate cause of aging.

Fast forward to 1984 when a new enzyme - telomerase - was discovered at the University of California. It results in the addition of new base pairs to telomeres thus lengthening them. This was exciting news because it led to speculation that if telomerase could be stimulated or pharmaceutically copied, it might be possible to lengthen our telomeres and hence our life spans.

Many experts though are not entirely convinced that telomere shortening is the ultimate explanation for aging, and favor further research. For example, in their 2008 publication titled "Telomeres and Aging" published in *Physiology Reviews*, Geraldine Auber and Peter M. Landor noted in their introduction that "it is also clear that **many mysteries around telomeres and their function remain**." (emphasis added)

This would seem to indicate that telomere length alone is not a sole determinant of health or age. I don't mean to say telomere length has no role. I just point out there is evidence that telomere length alone is not a direct determinant.

It is interesting to speculate though, if longer telomeres might be the genetic basis for the association of young mothers with longevity. A woman is born with all the follicles (egg forming structures) in her ovaries she will ever have. Eggs released earlier in life will have undergone fewer cell divisions and should therefore have longer telomeres. Could this be the source of the young mother advantage?

Bottom Line

Putting all this together, it seems to me most likely that the multi-factorial thesis is best. We inherit a genetic pre-disposition toward or away from certain disease and aging processes. The long telomeres of healthy eggs from a young mother may be the source of the pre-disposition, but it might also be inherently high levels of the antioxidant enzymes, or a combination of the two. That pre-disposition likely gives all of us, on average, the ability to live into our eighties – as long as we eat nutrient-dense foods, don't over-eat, and live an active life. With exercise, dietary discretion, a young mother, and the right genetics, we just might be able to live to be a healthy hundred years old or more.

The bottom line in all of this is that of all the factors discussed above, which do we control? And the answer is diet and exercise. And this exciting new practice of Age Management Medicine can give you the critical tool - hormonal optimization - to get the greatest benefit from your dietary and exercise efforts.

What Can Be Done about Aging?

The good news is that the symptoms of aging can be addressed through hormonal optimization, the correct diet, and proper exercise. Unlike some of the claims of my anti-aging colleagues, there is no magic bullet, no simple cure. It takes a combined approach and it takes conscious effort. But it can be done.

We've all heard the diet and exercise message, loud 'n clear from every public health voice in existence. We've heard it from our personal physicians, from celebrities, and that source of sources, the day-time television talk show host. We've heard it from fad diet promoters, diet food manufacturers, and exercise equipment marketers. Many of us have tried myriad of the pitched options ourselves, but without any real or sustained success. No, there isn't a magic bullet, but with the right hormonal milieu, you can do something about the aging process, and it's very likely a good deal easier than you think. But we need current information to begin.

Diagnostics

In order to improve our health, especially in our later years, it is essential to know our starting point. The first step in that regard is to produce an in-depth health history with current symptoms and concerns. In addition to a pertinent family health history, this includes a discussion of past personal health, diet, activity level, sex life patterns, and how all of these have changed over time.

Baseline diagnostic studies include an extensive blood hormone panel, body composition analysis, and fitness testing.

Assessment of hormone levels, for both men and women, include growth hormone (typically its surrogate test: IGF-1), thyroid hormones, thyroid stimulating hormone, insulin level, DHEA, estrogen, total and free testosterone, and LH. Also included are baseline organ health status tests for blood sugar, cell counts, and kidney and liver function. For women, the panel also includes progesterone and FSH. And for men, a prostate-specific antigen is part of the panel.

Body composition is determined by use of a DXA scanner, a very low-dose X-ray instrument. The instrument has an array of emitters and on the opposite side an array of sensors. These pass over the entire body in concert. Bone, lean tissue, and fat inhibit the passage of X-rays to different extents, and this can be measured so that it can quantitate total body muscle, bone and fat mass, and also fat distribution, i.e. visceral versus subcutaneous fat. This helps diagnose obesity, sarcopenia, osteopenia or osteoporosis.

Fitness testing is accomplished by determining some measure of one's anaerobic threshold. As mentioned, normal daily metabolism is aerobic, that is, it uses oxygen. Oxidative or aerobic metabolism is our most efficient route to energy utilization. But when energy demand exceeds the ability to deliver oxygen or to mobilize glucose stores, our bodies switch to anaerobic metabolism to fill the gap. Anaerobic is far less efficient and produces fatigue rapidly. It can only be maintained for brief periods.

The heart rate at which one begins to burn energy anaerobically is called the anaerobic threshold (AT). It can serve as a marker of fitness status, and also as a training tool. Heart rate at AT is different for everyone so in order to personalize an exercise prescription, it is essential to learn your baseline – your starting point – before undertaking a new exercise program.

Hormonal Optimization

Hormonal optimization is returning hormone levels to where they were when we were in our twenties and thirties. This can be accomplished to a large degree through lifestyle changes or nutritional supplementation but direct hormonal supplementation is also sometimes required.

The first step, of course, is the diagnostics. Getting baseline blood hormone levels. How do we know though, what is a "normal" or "low" level?

If you sample the blood of a large number of healthy people, at any age, the result is not a single, specific "normal" level. Levels vary significantly between otherwise-healthy persons. What you find is a range of values that are compatible with good health. As with essentially all biological functions, there is a "normal" distribution of values that when displayed graphically, results in the typical bell shaped curve we've all seen with lots of results crowded around the average – common things occur commonly – and fewer numbers are out at the higher and lower ends of the range; uncommon things occur less commonly.

The "standard deviation" is a measure of how spread out are the individual values within the population. In a normal distribution, 95% of values will fall within two standard deviations of the average value, and this range is typically used in medicine to define the "normal range." In this scenario, 2.5% of healthy individuals will fall outside the normal range at the top and the bottom. This relationship and definitions hold roughly true of any analyte, that is, whatever is being measured, whether it be sodium, potassium, insulin or estrogen.

It should also be noted that normal ranges can vary slightly between different laboratories due to dif-ferences in the test methodology used, and also the population sampled to establish the normal range. It is therefore important, as best as possible, to use the same laboratory when following a value over time.

Hormonal Deficiency

In medicine, a hormonal deficiency is usually defined as a value falling below the lower limit of the normal range, sometimes also referred to as the reference range. If the normal range for testosterone for an adult male is approximately 250-1,000 (depending upon laboratory and method used) a value of 260 is considered normal and not deficient. But let's say the man with the 260 value is now aged sixty and that when he was twenty, his level was 990. There is very strong probability that man will be experiencing age-related symptoms of testosterone deficiency - hypogonadism - even though he is not technically deficient.

It turns out that when comparing blood levels to symptoms, there is a significant overlap between people in the lower third of the normal range of values and those with symptoms. The onset of symptoms does not always correlate precisely with the end of the "normal range." This is especially true for growth hormone blood levels.

Remember that "normal" ranges are established by sampling large numbers of "healthy" individuals. But what is the definition of healthy in those samples? Typically a man volunteering to be sampled for a testosterone normal range study would be asked about high blood pressure, heart disease, strokes, diabetes, kidney disease, liver disease, et cetera. But would he be asked about his frequency of nocturnal erections or intimacy with his spouse? A research volunteer also wouldn't likely be asked how his body composition had changed over the course of his life nor about his energy level. It's easy to see then how a hypogonadal man could easily be included in a normal range study, and why there are significant numbers of symptomatic men in the lower third of the normal range.

Hormonal optimization, then, is a different treatment philosophy than treating deficiencies. Hormonal optimization is intervening to bring blood hormone levels in symptomatic individuals with values in the lower third of the normal range up to the upper third of the range. Exactly how that is accomplished varies with the specific hormone and the wishes of the individual patient, but the concept is important to understand because it is one of the most significant ways that AMM differs from a more traditional medical practice.

We all know someone – or perhaps we have experienced it ourselves – that as we age, we know we need to eat better and exercise more, but our efforts to do so frequently fail. That is why, despite the media barrage of public service message announcements over fifty years, we still have an epidemic of obesity and diabetes.

A 2010 poll by the *Associated Press* found that Americans over forty-five are "more obese than other generations." In that survey, nearly two-thirds of the respondents said they were dieting and exercising, but over two-thirds also indicated they were overweight or obese.

While heart attack rates have come down, thank goodness, they are still the leading cause of death in the U.S. So why are our efforts not working? Hormones. Hormonal optimization is the key to success in diet and exercise plans but it still is practiced only by a small minority of physicians. I can't tell you how many male patients I've spoken to or seen who tell me, "My doctor checked my testosterone but it was fine." But when I checked his levels, he was in the lower third.

This is not to say that physicians aren't doing their job, it's that they are not schooled in the new intricacies of AMM. That's why most doctors treating women for peri- or post-menopausal symptoms don't even check blood hormone levels. They treat their patients based only on symptoms. But then what is to prevent the woman's levels from getting too high when treated? Hormone therapy, like any pharmacologic intervention, can have side effects, and these become more likely with an increased dosage. So how does one give appropriate care and minimize risk of side effects without blood levels? This is the specialty of the Age Management Medicine practitioner.

Achieving Optimal Hormone Status

Our optimal goal is to get good hormone levels up into the upper - or in the case of insulin down into the lower - third of the normal range, but not too high or low.

Elevated insulin levels are best addressed with diet and exercise. Plain and simple. It takes some dedication and work but heck, as I say to my patients, "You don't really want diabetes, do you?"

The vast majority of people, even symptomatic ones, do not need GH supplementation. They may benefit from increasing GH levels, but except for cases of significant deficiency, that can usually be accomplished without medication. As previously noted, a significant proportion of GH secretion occurs during slow wave sleep. Improving SWS improves GH secretion. In addition, there is a fairly predictable GH secretion pulse after high-intensity exercise. Sleep is improved in most older adults with melatonin supplementation which also just so happens to be an excellent antioxidant. And adding or increasing high-intensity exercise to a workout plan also aids in improving GH.

Among men, slow wave sleep can often be further enhanced by reducing the need to awake for urination. The prostate gland surrounds a portion of the urethra, the tube connecting the urinary bladder to the outside world. The prostate gland grows with age, and if it becomes large enough, it can impede urine flow through the urethra at the time of urination, resulting in incomplete emptying of the bladder. Incomplete emptying leads to a need for more frequent urination, including at night when it interrupts sleep. The sleep interruptions this creates contribute to a decline in GH secretion.

The growth of the prostate is promoted over a lifetime by testosterone and its metabolites, most notably DHT. There are medications that inhibit the metabolism of testosterone to DHT and thereby help minimize prostate growth. Unfortunately, they sometimes also inhibit libido as DHT is a strong libido promoter. But there are also plant-based products that limit prostate growth by limiting DHT entry into the gland. These products are in widespread use in Europe, and are also available here in the U.S. as a dietary supplement.

For men with elevated estrogen, there is an effective oral medication that is an inhibitor of aromatase and will minimize conversion of testosterone to estrogen.

For men with adequate total testosterone yet high SHBG resulting in low levels of free or bioavailable hormone, there is an herbal product that can help. An extract of the root competes for the testosterone binding site on SHBG. With more herbal root molecules attached to the binding protein, there is less room for SHBG to gobble up testosterone. More testosterone remains unbound, free and active. For those with low total and free testosterone however, this is unlikely to be of benefit on its own, and hormonal supplementation may be required.

Testosterone has a role for women as well. Blood testosterone levels are the major determinant of libido. Though women make predominantly estrogen, a small proportion is converted via aromatase to testosterone, though at much lower levels than men. But those low levels play a significant role in libido. It is easily supplemented with topical cream. It can be applied to many skin sites but when applied directly to the clitoris, also helps improve sensitivity and often the quality of the sexual experience and helping attain orgasm.

Women open to post-menopausal hormone replacement now have the option of bioidentical hormones rather than the horse estrogen and synthetic progestins of the past. Early data indicate bioidentical hormones are effective and also likely safer than older preparations.

Results from Hormonal Optimization

Recall that the maximum benefit from AMM is achieved when hormonal optimization, diet, and exercise are combined. Hormonal optimization is excellent for symptomatic relief. But for true health improvement, optimization is only a tool to allow us to make even greater health and longevity strides through diet and exercise. That said, the symptomatic improvements can be dramatic.

For women, the most noticeable change is usually a

cessation of hot flashes, a particularly unsettling meno-pausal symptom. Men and women both experience an improved energy level for all of life's activities; for their families, their careers, and their personal pursuits.

Better sleep leads to a sense of improved general health as well as less perceived stress and anxiety. Less moodi-ness, irritability, angst, anger, and relationship dif-ficulties are prominent for some. A positive outlook returns.

Libido is generally noticeably improved with increased desire and also frequency of intimacy. Most people with optimized health enjoy an improved quality of their sexual experience. Men have more frequent and better quality erection, plus a better climax. Women enjoy less dryness, more sensitivity, and an enhanced ability to achieve orgasm. And these can be attained with local non-estrogen therapies for those who have an objection to systemic estrogen therapy.

With appropriate diet and exercise, both sexes can lose substantial body fat, particularly visceral fat. Not only does this help with improved disease risk factors such as blood pressure, cholesterol, and inflammation, but it also promotes better self image, confidence, and overall happiness. For some couples it may help relieve a point of contention in a relationship. For men with erectile dysfunction related to high blood pressure, weight loss can improve blood pressure and erectile function.

Again, with diet and exercise, muscle mass is improved. This promotes better resting metabolic rate and energy consumption, helping to maintain weight loss. It promotes a more positive self-image and improves exercise and athletic tolerance, performance and recovery. Risk of future falls and fractures is diminished. Bone mass is improved, again reducing fracture risk and its associated morbidity and mortality.

When hormonal optimization is combined with stress/anxiety-reduction strategies, the mood improvements mentioned above can be pronounced. Libido and sexual function changes are also more positively affected. A positive outlook and happiness can return.

Exercise

With hormones optimized, our bodies are well equipped to benefit from exercise. Ample data exist that exercise helps reduce disease risk factors as well as improve personal perception of general overall health status.

Weight Loss and Control

Exercise can help prevent excess weight gain, maintain healthy weight, and improve fat loss. Exercise burns calories above baseline. The more intense the activity, the more calories are burned. Burning more calories than are taken in can contribute to weight loss. Balancing calories burned with those consumed helps maintain healthy weight. Exercise improves glucose sensitivity, lessening the risk of diabetes. It improves cardiovascular fitness and athletic performance which allows even more and better exercise.

During exercise, there is an increase in oxygen uptake (VO_2) to support the increased energy need. After exercise of sufficient intensity and duration, VO_2 does not return to resting levels immediately, but may remain elevated above resting for some period of time. This phenomenon is called excess post-exercise oxygen consumption or EPOC. This typically lasts about one hour but may be as long as several hours. Little or no EPOC is seen with low-intensity, short-duration exercise but more is seen by increasing intensity and duration. Smaller increased increments in intensity produce greater results than the same incremental increase in duration. Working harder has more effect than working longer.

Supramaximal exercise is exercise that goes beyond the maximal rate of muscular oxygen consumption, at which point the body no longer creates energy using oxygen, but rather switches to anaerobic metabolism. Supramaximal exercise is high intensity exercise so it should not be surprising that it induces more EPOC.

Muscle Mass and Strength

Resistance exercise helps build muscle mass and endurance and also contributes to EPOC. Muscle mass burns more calories at rest than any other tissue. Maintaining muscle mass and strength helps reduce the risk of frailty and falls with older age.

Exercise Fights Disease/Promotes Health

Exercise level and obesity are independent risk factors for vascular diseases. In other words, no matter what your weight, being active boosts high-density lipoprotein (HDL), or "good" cholesterol and decreases unhealthy triglycerides. It also improves insulin sensitivity, which decreases risk of cardiovascular diseases and Type 2 diabetes. Regular physical activity can help prevent and/or manage a wide range of health problems including stroke, metabolic syndrome, Type 2 diabetes, depression, arthritis, falls, dementia and Alzheimer's disease. And these last, dementia and Alzheimer's are worth emphasizing. There are very few interventions known to help reduce risk for these devastating ailments. But among them, the most well studied and most effective is exercise.

Exercise Improves Mood

A workout at the gym or a brisk thirty-minute walk can help relieve stress and improve mood. Physical activity stimulates brain chemicals that may leave you feeling happier and more relaxed. You may also feel better about your appearance with regular exercise, which can boost your confidence and improve your self-esteem.

Exercise Boosts Energy Levels

Regular physical activity improves muscle strength and boosts endurance. Exercise and physical activity deliver oxygen and nutrients to your tissues, and help your cardiovascular system work more efficiently. And when your heart and lungs work more efficiently, you have more energy to go about your daily activities.

Exercise Can Mean Better Sleep

Regular physical activity can help you fall asleep faster and deepen your sleep. And we've previously discussed the value of sleep in avoiding fatigue, stress, and anxiety, and in boosting natural growth hormone secretion.

Exercise Can Mean a Better Sex Life

Regular physical activity can leave you feeling energized and looking better, which can have a positive effect on your sex life. But there's more to it than that. Regular physical activity can also lead to enhanced arousal for women. And men who exercise regularly are less likely to have problems with erectile dysfunction than are men who don't. Remember that heart health is penis health!

What Is the "Best Exercise?"

That exercise is healthy and helpful is clear. The list of conditions that can be prevented or minimized by exercise includes cardiovascular disease, stroke, high blood pressure, Type 2 diabetes, osteoporosis, obesity, colon cancer, breast cancer, anxiety, depression, and cognitive function.

But there are so many mixed messages in popular culture and the news media about what type of exercise is best. Though there is no "one size fits all approach" to exercise, what is absolutely clear is that both resistance training and cardiovascular exercise are needed; resistance training to build or maintain muscle mass, and cardiovascular for fat loss and maintenance of good body composition.

There are three variables in any workout regimen:

frequency, intensity, and duration. Of the three, frequency is definitely the most important when starting from scratch. For someone leading a sedentary lifestyle, just walking briskly for a half-hour three days a week can make a measurable difference in body composition and insulin sensitivity. I call that the couch potato workout, but warn that for it to have effect, it must be a consistent minimum three days and a consistent half-hour each session. For the best results I recommend greater frequency, intensity, and duration.

The standard public health message for fifty years now has been the "long slow distance" approach to cardiovascular fitness exercise. That is, low intensity for a longer duration. That is, in fact, effective for improving cardiovascular fitness. It is significantly less effective, however, for fat loss. Fat loss can be better achieved with higher intensity levels. And higher intensity levels can require shorter durations to achieve that goal.

The magnitude of EPOC is higher on average for men than for women, but this difference is related largely to men having a higher average body mass. Where men and women have equal body mass, the magnitude of EPOC is the same for both.

One of the guiding principles of AMM is to personalize/customize exercise regimens as best as possible for each patient. What constitutes low, moderate, and high intensity is different for each individual, of course. Therein lies the need for – and the value of – the objective diagnostics.

Fitness testing on a treadmill or bicycle with determination of anaerobic threshold is essential to customize an exercise prescription. And also, each patient should first be assessed for any possible contraindications to exercise testing such as unstable angina or a tendency to lose consciousness. These variables are why it is not possible to give specific recommendations to all readers of this book. Generally, for my patients, I recommend this weekly regimen:

Three to six days total of cardiovascular fitness training;

One to two days of high-intensity intervals (HIIT), one-minute bursts of supramaximal, anaerobic exercise;

The day following an HIIT day should be a recovery day which can be either rest or a low-intensity cardiovascular training of a short duration;

Twenty to thirty minutes total time for HIIT days to include up to four, one-minute intervals followed periods after each high intensity interval; recovery is at low intensity;

Two to three days of moderate intensity;

Minimum thirty to maximum sixty minutes for moderate intensity training;

Three days per week minimum of resistance training.

Stretching or yoga essentially every day but certainly not less than five days per week.

Resistance Training

Resistance training can be accomplished with hand weights, resistance bands, free weights or weight machines. My comments below relate to weight training, but in a customized plan for those who don't enjoy gyms and weights, I also put together workouts using only hand weights or bands.

Resistance training, too, needs customization but is more difficult to objectively assess. Fitness magazines and the internet are brimming with articles proclaiming that their method is best. As in cardiovascular fitness training, frequency, and intensity are important and can be varied depending upon the patient's goals, motivation, and available time to commit.

As to frequency, a whole body workout at each exercise session, three days per week is sufficient to contribute to EPOC and build muscle mass. But it won't make a bodybuilder out of anyone. Then again, that isn't our goal. Our goal is simply to increase total body muscle mass.

For those seeking more pronounced results, resistance training six days per week, rotating muscle groups, and never going more than ninety-six hours without exercising any single muscle group is much more effective.

But to insist on that level of commitment from the average patient is to invite failure. Most folks just aren't that committed. Even though they would like to do the work, they have time constraints and other factors in their everyday lives that need attention.

In resistance training, intensity is the volume of work done. Volume is weight-times-repetitions-times-sets of each exercise. In AMM, the goal of resistance training is muscle mass gain. There is sound scientific evidence that the best results for mass building are at three sets of 65% to 85% of an individual's maximum resistance for that movement, performed for ten repetitions. Though that may be most effective, it is certainly not the only way.

Typically, Nautilus-type weight machine circuits provide only two sets for each muscle group. But they are very time efficient and favored by many. So for those who wish to use a training circuit, I typically recommend keeping weight to about 75% of maximum and doing fifteen repetitions.

(For those of you not familiar with the term, a circuit means working out using a select variety of different exercise machines. Most of the machines can be set to variable strength requirements, enabling you to set an appropriate exercise level, and to adjust it over time.)

As an experiment, let's calculate a rough estimate of the volume of exercise for these two approaches. Doing three sets of ten at 85% (with a maximum of 100), volume is 3x85x10=2550. For a circuit the volume is 2x75x15 = 2250. The volumes are similar though there is some advantage to the three sets of ten at 85%.

Your maximum is the maximum weight that you can lift or move for one repetition, i.e., a single lift or move. This should not be attempted with free weights like barbells without professional assistance. And doing maximal weights even on a machine carries some risk of injury. So I tell my patients to estimate it. If you can't reach eight repetitions, the weight is too high. If you can do fifteen without fatigue, it's too low.

Optimum Diet

Dietary goals for AMM are:

> Adequate, but not excess, calories

> Adequate protein

> Minimize insulin

> Adequate antioxidant intake

In contradistinction to the standard typical healthy diet pyramid which rests on a base of grains, a carbohydrate-controlled or low glycemic diet pyramid would have as its base, lean meats along with ample fruits and vegetables. Grains would reside at the tip on the top. This is often also referred to as the hunter-gatherer, Paleolithic or caveman diet as it mimics the typical diet of our forebears and how we evolved. Studies of those ancient peoples show a near absence of the chronic degenerative diseases that have become the death knell for so many of our age. Pre-agricultural humans were never obese!

It really is quite simple to achieve these goals. The science isn't complicated. But the lifestyle changes may be difficult for some. The basics are simple:

Don't over-eat. I'm not a fan of calorie counting. Its cumbersome and annoying. It is often a source of failure when starting a new diet. I think most people know when they are full. I tell my patients to eat until they are full, then stop. Despite what our mothers told us, the plight of starving children in poor countries is not improved if we clean our plates.

Avoid high- glycemic index foods. As discussed in the section about insulin levels and dietary intake, this typically is anything white: SUGAR, white bread, white rice, potatoes (sweet potatoes are all right), et cetera. Eating whole, non-processed foods and avoiding pre-pared packaged foods goes a long way toward accomplishing this goal.

Eat adequate protein. For years the recommendation has been to eat 0.8grams per kg of body weight. More recent research though indicates that for physically-active adults – and we want our patients active – 1.6 to 1.8 grams per kg of their weight is more effective and appropriate. The problem is, most people can absorb only 25 to 35 grams at a single meal. For folks who weigh over 170 pounds, it is difficult to eat enough protein in three meals according to this formula. For these people I recommend snacking between their main meals; that is, mid-morning and mid-afternoon low-calorie, high-protein snacks are recommended.

Adequate antioxidant intake. There is good evidence that it is possible to eat enough fruits and vegetables daily to meet our needs. The National Cancer Institute, the American Cancer Society, and the American Heart Association all agree with that conclusion. They actually go one step further and come out against the use of antioxidant dietary supplements.

But how much fruit and vegetable intake constitutes "adequate" fruits and vegetables? According to the American Heart Association, it is **4.5 cups per day**! Have you ever laid out all at once, four and a half cups of produce? Food preferences aside, the sheer volume is daunting for all but the most committed. The average American nowadays works, cares for children, is sometimes also caring for an elderly parent or ailing spouse, and, if that American is one of my patients, he is also making time for exercise and fitness. Trying to fit in the time to prepare vegetables three times a day might not be entirely realistic. Especially if one throws food preferences into the mix. Not everyone enjoys vegetables, any vegetables, and for these reasons I do, in fact, recommend antioxidant supplements to my patients.

I concur with the National Center for Complementary

and Alternative Medicine that supplements should not be used as a substitute for eating fresh fruits and vegetables. It is important to make every effort to consume as much fruit and vegetables (and whole grains) as possible. But a nutritional "supplement," used in exactly that manner - as a supplement, not a replacement - can certainly increase the likelihood of optimum antioxidant intake. But how to do that?

Our bodies make our own non-enzymatic antioxidants, including glutathione, a three-amino acid chain that includes cysteine. Increasing dietary intake of cysteine can help us make more of our own glutathione, which itself, is not well absorbed in the intestinal tract. Dietary sources include meats, red peppers, garlic, onions, broccoli, Brussels sprouts, whole oats, wheat germ, and whey protein. Dietary supplementation with n-acetyl-cysteine is also effective at boosting glutathione levels.

Melatonin, discussed previously in the context of sleep, also possesses a powerful antioxidant capacity and may scavenge a variety of ROS. Supplements are readily available over the counter.

Two-amino acid chain peptides, histidine dipeptides, are a family of compounds synthesized in the brain and skeletal muscles, two tissues particularly susceptible to oxidants. These compounds, including carnosine, possess strong antioxidant capabilities. The amino acids found in carnosine are found in high quantity in beef, pork, poultry, and fish. Dietary supplements are also available.

Dietary antioxidants such as the majority that are found in fruits and vegetables can be absorbed as such and do, in fact, help our bodies control possible damage secondary to free radicals and other reactive oxygen species. A diet rich in fruits and vegetables provides ample doses of exogenous antioxidants.

Vitamin C is an efficient antioxidant.

The family of tocopherol antioxidants are eight naturally-occurring members of the vitamin E family. The most effective form is d-alpha tocopherol. Although all possess antioxidant activity, the d-alpha - tocopherol is considered the most effective as the others are not retained and absorbed as well in body tissues. But the tocotrienol group may also have cholesterol-lowering properties, and some supplements specifically include these.

The AMM goal then, is to ensure maximum production of endogenous (self-produced) antioxidants as well as having our patients consume and supplement with plant based antioxidants.

There are so many supplement products on the market with new ones introduced regularly. It seems that nearly every week a new super food is trumpeted as the newest and best source of antioxidants for our health. They all seem to claim the highest ever ORAC value. ORAC (oxygen radical absorbance capacity) is the most commonly used laboratory test of antioxidant capacity of foods. It's a fairly simple matter to test foods in the laboratory for their antioxidant capacity. In order for that food to enhance our body's antioxidant capacity though, it must first be digested and absorbed.

Laboratory measurements of a food's ORAC do not necessarily indicate how that will translate to ORAC in our blood. Some foods are better absorbed than others, and there is a variance in cultures and individuals. There are data on absorption rates of different high ORAC foods, but also, once eaten and absorbed, food elements are metabolized and the metabolic process may alter a food's antioxidant capacity.

The net result is that ORAC claims are not a particularly good way of assessing a food's or supplement's nutritional value. In the absence of a well-validated test for assessing antioxidant capacity, I think it best to simply look for supplements that (1) are food-based and (2) include a mixture of both fruits and vegetables. They should include both multiple fruits and multiple vegetables to ensure adequate variety.

Among the vegetable sources, a food-based supplement should include at a minimum, at least one cruciferous vegetable such as broccoli, cauliflower, kale, and cabbage, plus lycopene from tomatoes. Among the fruits, a mixture of berries is likely to have significant antioxidant content. Pomegranate, apple skin or whole apples, and green tea are good as well.

An effective supplement that is not specifically food based is alpha-lipoic acid (LA) which is a naturally-occurring sulphur containing short-chain fatty acid. There is growing evidence that orally supplied LA may elicit a unique set of biochemical activities with potential therapeutic value against a host of biologic insults. So although I recommend it principally as an antioxidant, it is also clear that it may well have numerous other health benefits.

Selenium also has antioxidant activity and is now typically included in most multivitamins. At high levels though, it may have toxic effects. "If some is good, more is better" certainly does not apply here, so don't overdo selenium.

In summary, it is possible to obtain adequate amounts of exogenous antioxidants from dietary sources. Adequate intake though is in the range of 4.5 cups of mixed fruits and vegetables every day. If that volume of dietary intake is not practical, the use of food-based supplements of mixed fruits and vegetables is entirely reasonable, and perhaps even desirable, depending upon one's dietary preferences. Selenium along with vitamins C and E are safe and effective. And it is certainly reasonable but not necessary to add other supplements as discussed.

In this discussion of food supplements I should also make note of marine fish body oil and its active ingredients, the omega-3 fatty acids, EPA and DHA. Though they are not antioxidants per se, they have multiple beneficial effects. First and foremost they are extremely effective at reducing triglyceride, the most significant bad fat contributing to vascular disease. In addition though, they are anti-inflammatory and there is increasing evidence they may prevent and/or slow the progression of arthritis and age related cognitive decline. I strongly recommend everyone take a fish oil supplement. But take care to be certain that it is mercury- free.

Conclusion

Thanks to the efforts of an army of late 19th and early 20th century scientists and engineers, many humans have been saved from early-age disability and death from the infectious plagues of the past. Further, late 20th century researchers discovered the mechanisms behind some of the most debilitating and lethal chronic degenerative diseases, and highlighted some measurable aging conditions; those being largely hormonal and metabolic. We also now have the means to objectively quantify the changes in our aging parameters.

Now it's up to us. We have the tools to live better, longer. But it takes personal health data analysis, and it requires personal effort. It is my hope that this book has helped to further your understanding of aging and to encourage you to seek the guidance and care of physicians and other health care professionals who can guide you to a healthier, more functional, and happier journey that we all take. Where it will end we know not. But there is much that we can do to control the quality of the journey.

Be well.

Live Better Longer

Some More Thoughts

The Women's Health Initiative

Postmenopausal hormone replacement therapy (HRT) for women was the norm for many years in the U.S. and in the developed countries of western and northern Europe. Typically the main goal of the therapy was cessation of hot flashes. Of all the manifestations of the menopause, hot flashes seemed to be the most bothersome. For many women though, loss of libido and sexual dysfunction were also big motivators for therapy.

Doctors, of course, had their own motivations. In addition to their patient's desires, they looked to decrease osteoporosis and fracture risk, and also to cardiovascular (CV) disease risk for their patients.

Prior to menopause, women's CV disease risk is lower than for men. But afterwards, women's risk catches up. Hormone replacement therapy can help reduce that risk.

It should be noted in this regard though, that female hormone replacement therapy is not without risk. It was discovered early on that replacement estrogen alone – without concomitant progesterone administration – greatly increased the risk of developing endometrial type uterine cancer. Simultaneous administration of estrogen and progesterone, though, eliminated this risk, and we now no longer see any excess cases of endometrial carcinoma.

Over time though, a slight increase in breast cancer risk was seen. Since this was slight, it was thought to be more than offset by the decreased risk of fractures and their associated morbidity and mortality, and also the lowered risk of cardiovascular events.

About a decade ago though, initial results of a newer research effort examining the use of HRT – it was called the Women's Health Initiative (WHI) – were published, and its findings ran contrary to prior data and the accepted convention described above. Four treatment groups were studied. The results were complex and difficult to summarize, but the most significant finding was about women who had not had a hysterectomy; those who still had their uterus and thus the risk of endometrial uterine cancer needed to be treated with both estrogen and a progestin. As expected, this group registered a reduction in fractures. But there was also an increase in cardiovascular events. This finding was quite shocking because it ran contrary to forty years of experience.

The WHI had significant flaws though, with regard to its finding of an increase in CV disease. First, it has been long known that the potential beneficial effects of HRT are best achieved when begun in the immediate or early post-menopausal period. The longer after menopause HRT is begun, the less likely women are to benefit. The WHI enrolled women in the study who were as old as seventy-nine. The average age of women entering the study was sixty-three; well after the typical onset of menopause and not typical of women for whom HRT is normally considered. And it is an age far more prone to CV disease based on age alone.

Second, if the age issue alone weren't enough, roughly a third of the WHI enrollees were obese, and a similar proportion had high blood pressure, both of which are risk factors for CV disease.

Given the older ages of the participants and the high rate of other obesity and high blood pressure, it was clear to most medical observers that the WHI greatly over-estimated the risk of adverse CV events. But the published results generated substantial negative press coverage for HRT, and as a result, there was a dramatic change in the perception of the value of HRT among women despite contrary evidence published both before and since.

The net result was a complete turnaround in the perception of HRT and the choices women had been making. A substantial proportion of women then on HRT discontinued the therapy, and a majority of newly-menopausal women opted not to begin it at all. As a result of the questionable research and the unquestioning media, I think many women have suffered needlessly from menopausal symptoms because of fears conjured up by the initial WHI findings.

On another front, the WHI also found the previously-documented and expected increase in breast cancer. But after publication of the WHI, this seemed less worthy of tolerating in the absence of one of the main supposed beneficial effects, reduced CV risk.

The baseline lifetime risk for breast cancer in the United States is stated by the National Cancer Institute (NCI) and American Cancer Society (ACS) as about one-in-eight or about 12% of women by age ninety-five. This assumes though that all women live to at least ninety-five when in fact, the life expectancy for American women is roughly eighty. Since the risk of breast cancer increases dramatically with age, the WHI's projection based on age ninety-five appears to be a significant over-estimation.

The National Surgical Adjuvant Breast and Bowel Project (NSABP) is a clinical trials cooperative group that has more than fifty years experience designing and conducting clinical trials on the way breast cancer is treated, and, more recently, prevented.

Based on NSABP data, the risk of a fifty-year-old woman with no family history of breast cancer and other risk factors in the low range would have a risk of developing breast cancer at some time over the rest of her life of about 6%. If she had no family history but had other risk factors in the higher range, her risk would be about 11%. The midpoint is about 8%. These numbers seem more accurate to me than the theoretical calculations of the NCI and ACS. Regardless, the point is that there is a baseline risk of breast cancer even in women who do not use HRT, and to reiterate, I suggest that baseline figure is around 8% of women living to eighty years old. What we would like to know is how much that risk is increased by HRT.

Returning to the WHI study and increased breast cancer risk of approximately one quarter, the increase they saw on top of a baseline of 8% translates to a new risk of roughly 10%, or two points higher. So, using HRT would increase a woman's risk of breast cancer from 8% to 10% That is not insignificant, but it is also vastly less than how most women and the news media understood the WHI data. I even had one recent prospective patient tell me that her understanding from WHI was that "essentially all the women got breast cancer." And she was a highly-educated and intelligent woman.

So contrary to early reports, it is now clear the HRT not only eliminates symptoms, but if begun in the early postmenopausal period, helps reduce risk for osteoporosis/bone fractures, heart disease, strokes and dementia

Progestins

With respect to that increased risk of breast cancer seen in the WHI and other studies, all of the early studies were conducted using conjugated equine (horse) estrogens (CEE) and progestins, not bio-identical proges-terone. Progestins are synthetic progesterone. When it was discovered in the 1930s that one of progesterone's effects is that it suppresses ovulation during pregnancy, efforts began to use progesterone as birth control.

It was soon discovered that progesterone identical to the naturally-occurring variety could be synthesized in the laboratory. The problem was that it was only very poorly absorbed when administered orally, and it produced substantial local irritation when given by intramuscular injection. This then lead to the ultimate development of synthetic progesterone compounds collectively known as progestins.

These compounds were approved for use in Europe much sooner than in the U.S. where they went into widespread use in the 1960s.

In the WHI, one branch of the study included women who had previously had a hysterectomy and so were able to receive estrogen alone without a progestin. This group did not show the increase in breast cancer seen in the combined therapy group thus indicating the increased risk may have resulted from the synthetic progestin, not the estrogen. Other studies have found similar results.

Bio-identical progesterone also had been in use in Europe longer than here in the US. Research studies there have indicated a lower or even absent risk of breast cancer in women using bio-identical progesterone. It is a bit early to be able to say with certainty, but I believe long term follow-up studies of women using bio-identical estrogen and progesterone therapy will show little or no increased risk of breast cancer.

Testosterone for Men

There is ample evidence that higher blood testosterone levels are not related to prostate cancer. There is a risk though, that testosterone therapy can promote the growth of pre-existing prostate cancer. However, the magnitude of this risk appears low, and also is very likely confined almost entirely to men who have previously been treated for metastatic cancer (where the disease has spread beyond the prostate) with testosterone lowering or blocking drugs. Men with known prostate cancer not treated with such measures have been given testosterone therapy without an increase in recurrence rate or poor outcome. Dr. Abraham Morgentaler, a urologist and expert in testosterone therapy has said, "I believe the best summary about the risk of prostate cancer from testosterone therapy ... is as follows:

> "Low blood levels of testosterone do not protect against prostate cancer and, indeed, may increase the risk.

> "High blood levels of testosterone do not increase the risk of prostate cancer.

"Treatment with testosterone does not increase the risk of prostate cancer, even among men who are already at high risk for it."

From all of my studies and experience, as a physician I feel very comfortable prescribing testosterone for my patients with symptoms of hypogonadism who have no current evidence of prostate cancer.

Growth Hormone

Though GH has been used for decades in children with congenital GH deficiency without any evidence of an increased incidence of cancer, there is a theoretical concern that since GH promotes tissue growth. Hence, it might promote the growth of pre-existing malignant tumors. For this reason, its use is considered not indicated in persons with a past history of malignancy.

Telomeres

Imagine browsing the Health and Wellness section of your favorite local or online bookstore. You might be leafing through a just-published book on longevity. In it you discover that "it is now possible for you to extend your life expectancy beyond one hundred years to one hundred-twenty or more (**perhaps indefinitely**) …all without having to worry about life-threatening conditions like cancer, heart disease… dementia…" Browsing further you learn that "Living cells, including human ones, **never have to die**..." (emphasis added) These claims, among many others, are featured in a book published in 2011; it is a perfect example of the contrast mentioned earlier between anti-aging and Age Management physicians.

These are bold claims that neither myself nor anyone else can refute. It's hard to refute a claim that something is "possible." But I would say that it is not yet supported by a preponderance of the scientific evidence. I mention this here because you may have read the book, or may at least be familiar with its central theme which is the importance of the genetic structures called telomeres, which were previously covered in the chapter on basic biologic processes. I reprise it here because that book also proposed a longevity strategy involving efforts to lengthen telomeres.

A Northern California biotechnology firm has developed a non-FDA approved, non-prescription dietary supplement derived from the Chinese herb astragulus purported to lengthen telomeres. It is marketed to consumers specifically through their own network of anti-aging physicians. It is purported to promote telomerase activity and lengthen telomeres and with them, supposedly, life span. This was exciting news indeed. Easy access to an over the counter dietary supplement that could extend human life would be almost certainly widely-attractive and, potentially, remarkably remunerative.

The product has been subjected to only a single scientific inquiry published in a peer reviewed scientific journal. The results were encouraging:

> Cells grown in tissue culture with the proprietary supplement showed lengthening of their telomeres.

> Immune cells from the blood of volunteers taking the supplement showed a reduction in the percentage of circulating immune cells with critically short telomeres. (However, there was no overall average lengthening of immune cell telomeres in the total population of cells.)

> The blood of volunteers previously infected with CMV (cytomegalovirus) taking the supplement showed a reduction in the proportion of senescent immune cells.

Yes, these are mostly encouraging results, but you should know that there were problems with the study. First , understand that there is a difference between laboratory findings (in vitro) and results from testing in a living human (in vivo). Indeed, it is a not infrequent in medical science that in vitro findings cannot be replicated in vivo. So it must be kept in mind that the findings in tissue culture cells treated in the laboratory, as in the study mentioned above, have not as yet been replicated in cells taken from treated humans.

Secondly, the study had no control group. The

researchers studied treated volunteers. A study needs to include a group examined on the same issue but having taken only a placebo, instead of the focus drug. Otherwise, there is no way of knowing if the changes in the treated group might have resulted from something other than the treatment.

Say, for example, the results came from normal cyclical or random variation in the number of senescent cells or those with critically short telomeres. It may be possible that those numbers change periodically without treatment, and that timing was the true reason for the lower numbers seen after treatment.

Third, the product had only been tested on peripheral blood immune system cells. Other cells and tissues had not been studied.

Maybe most significant is that the findings have not been replicated. The ability of other, unrelated scientists to replicate earlier findings is a critical part of the scientific method. It has not yet been happened in this instance.

And then there is this...four of the five authors have disclosed (appropriately) financial interests in the success of the product. Two of the authors disclosed in addition, their personal involvement as subjects in the research study.

What I have presented here is not by any means an exhaustive review of the scientific literature on the role of telomeres in aging and disease. I present these issues only to make the point that the biochemical processes involved in telomere biology are complex, incompletely understood, and that in the absence of a more complete understanding, such grand proclamations of immortality seem to me, at least at present, unwarranted. Because even if telomere length is the single most significant determinant of the genetic component to aging, my earlier examination of that topic makes it clear that we can negate whatever genetic advantage we are granted through bad choices. Sedentary lifestyle and obesity trump genetics, and long telomeres. Diet and exercise - correct diet and exercise - still matter and hormonal optimization is still an effective tool for enabling good body composition.

Calorie Restriction

Few therapies have been found that consistently extend the life span of multiple species. Calorie restriction (CR), the reduction in the total volume of dietary intake while maintaining sufficient micro-nutrient (vitamins and minerals) intake, is a notable exception. Studies in the 1930s established the effectiveness of CR for extending the life span of rats. Subsequent studies have demonstrated that sustained reductions in calorie intake can increase maximum life span in a wide range of species. CR increases longevity of rodents, fish, invertebrates and in some, but not all flies. Most notably, maintaining mice and rats from a young age at 20% to 40% below average unrestricted food intake extends life span significantly beyond their free feeding brethren in the control group.

The theory is that physiologic responses to insufficient calories represent an adaptive response to food scarcity. In order for it to be passed on evolutionarily, a trait must provide a reproductive advantage over those without the trait. The biggest reproductive advantage of course is to survive long enough to reproduce at all, or to reproduce more successfully. So in order to be passed on o the next generation, a trait must be advantageous. So goes the theory.

But not all laboratory animal studies have found a longevity extension in response to CR. CR does not increase life span in butterflies, some insects and rotifers, multi-cellular aquatic organisms.

Studies in higher order mammals have had mixed results. Rhesus monkeys are non-human primates that have long been used in research as human surrogates. In a study published in 2003, CR was reported to extend life span in Rhesus monkeys. But that project studied only eight monkeys, and subsequent studies have not reproduced the finding in animals followed for as long as seventeen years; thus a possible benefit in non-human primates remains a very open question.

These are just a few examples to make the point that the relationship between CR and increased longevity is not universal. There are plenty of exceptions. This is an important point because if it is a universal, or near universal phenomenon, then it would seem logical that CR would likely be effective in humans as well.

Most human studies have not been continued for extended periods. Also, with few exceptions the human data to date are largely derived from dietary reduction specifically for weight loss among overweight or obese persons, which of course brings about measurable health benefits from weight loss alone and not necessarily specifically from CR.

To better address this question, the National Institute on Aging (NIA) recently funded a multi-site human clinical trial to assess the effects of two years of CR (around 25% restriction) in non-obese, healthy people. Preliminary results indicate that many of the metabolic and physiologic responses observed in rodents and monkeys are reproducible in humans. These include reduced total body weight, along with reductions in subcutaneous fat, visceral fat, more insulin sensitivity, improved blood cholesterol levels, reduced energy expenditure, and core body temperature.

But the reduced energy expenditure and lower body temperature come at the expense of reduced lean body mass. Muscle mass is lost. Assuming this type of dietary restraint is sustainable beyond the short term, one might expect these physiological changes to predict a decrease in age-related disease in the long run.

But most evolutionary biologists are not convinced these types of physiologic changes would have provided a selective advantage to early humans. For organisms unable to escape their environment during times of food scarcity, one can see how decreased energy consumption and lower body mass that allowed survival on lower food quantity would convey a survival advantage. But for nomadic organisms like humans, the ability to travel to more hospitable environs might obviate the need to hunker down, slow down, and rest. And if, as it appears, mobility was evolving man's survival strategy, the changes of CR may not be adaptive in the long term. It could be that diminished resting metabolic rate – slowing down because of restricted calorie intake – may be associated with a slow decline to frailty and death.

Despite this, some of the results – improved cholesterol and better insulin sensitivity, for example – are promising and there are many dedicated adherents to the CR theory of longevity. Most doctors and researchers though, believe that a substantial majority of folks would prefer not to restrict their diet in the presence of an abundant food supply.

Protein restriction (PR) and intermittent fasting (IF), two dietary restriction techniques that are similar to CR but do not require a reduction in overall calorie intake every day, are also under scientific investigation to determine their value in anti-aging.

Despite these investigations, currently, there are no

known dietary or pharmacologic interventions proven to substantially slow the aging process in humans, including CR. This doesn't mean it has been proven ineffective. What it means is that data proving that it is effective are lacking. And part of the reason for that is the same set of logistical and ethical problems mentioned in the earlier discussion of the genetics of aging: the relatively long life span of humans that makes accurate and meaningful follow-up difficult, both medically and ethically.

Glossary

aerobic metabolism - oxygen-requiring metabolism of sugars and fatty acids to CO_2 and H_2O.

amino acid - an organic compound containing at least one amino (nitrogen) group and one carboxyl (carbon) group.

base pair - association of two complementary nucleotides in a DNA molecule stabilized by chemical bonds between their base components. Adenine pairs with thymine (A ·T) and guanine pairs with cytosine (G ·C).

catalyst - a substance that enables a chemical reaction to proceed at a faster rate or under different conditions (as at a lower temperature) than otherwise possible.

carbohydrate - General term for carbon containing compounds that are the primary type of compound used for storing and supplying energy in animal cells.

cell - the smallest unit of life that carries out its own processes. The cell consists primarily of an outer membrane, which separates it from the environment; the genetic material (DNA), which encodes heritable information, and the cytoplasm, a complex solution of salts and other molecules.

cell membrane - The outer membrane of a cell, which separates it from the environment. Also called a plasma membrane.

chromosome - the structure that holds the genetic material consisting of a single, linear double-stranded DNA molecule and associated proteins.

DNA - deoxyribonucleic acid is the double-helix molecule holding the genetic information of organisms that, along with protein, composes the chromosomes.

enzyme - A biological catalyst. Most enzymes are proteins.

gene - Physical and functional unit of heredity, which carries information from one generation to the next. In molecular terms, it is the entire DNA sequence necessary for production of a functional protein.

glucose - Six-carbon sugar that is the primary metabolic fuel in most cells. The large glucose polymer, glycogen is used to store energy in animal cells.

glycogen - A very long, branched polysaccharide, composed exclusively of glucose units, that is the primary storage carbohydrate in animal cells. It is found primarily in liver and muscle cells.

hormone - General term for any extracellular substance that induces specific responses in target cells. Hormones coordinate the growth and metabolic activities of various cells, tissues, and organs in multicellular organisms.

in vitro - Denoting a reaction or process taking place in a laboratory environment, outside an organism.

in vivo - In an intact cell or organism.

insulin - A protein hormone produced in the pancreas that stimulates uptake of glucose into liver, muscle and fat cells, and helps to regulate blood glucose levels.

lipid - Any organic molecule that is insoluble in water but is soluble in non-charged organic solvents (think fat). Lipids are chains of fatty acids and are found in cell and nuclear membranes.

macromolecule - Any large, usually polymeric molecule (e.g., a protein, nucleic acid, polysaccharide) with a molecular mass greater than a certain cutoff.

membrane -- Semi-fluid structure which bounds all cells, and partitions the interior of cells. It consists primarily of two lipid layers, with proteins "dissolved" in the lipids.

metabolism - The sum of all chemical reactions producing energy in cells.

neuron (nerve cell) - Any of the impulse-conducting cells of the nervous system.

nuclear membrane - The double membrane which surrounds the cell nucleus. It has many pores in its surface which regulate the flow of large compounds into and out of the nucleus.

nucleus - Large membrane-bounded organelle in cells that contains DNA organized into chromosomes. The cell's control center.

organ - Structures made of two or more tissues which function as an integrated unit e.g. the heart, kidneys, liver, stomach.

oxidation - The loss of electrons or hydrogen ion in a chemical reaction.

polymer - Any large molecule composed of multiple identical or similar units (monomers) linked by chemical bonds.

protein - A linear polymer of amino acid sub units linked together in a specific sequence and usually containing more than 50 subunits. Proteins form the key structural elements in cells and participate in nearly all cellular activities.

polypeptide - Proteins are large polypeptides, and the two terms commonly are used interchangeably.

receptor - Any protein that binds a specific extracellular signaling molecule and then initiates a cellular response. Receptors for steroid hormones are located within the cell; receptors for water-soluble hormones, e.g., insulin, protein growth factors, and neurotransmitters are located in the plasma membrane exposed to the external medium.

stem cell - A self-renewing cell with multiple developmental potentials. A cell that hasn't yet decided what it is going to be when it grows up.

steroid - Any of numerous naturally occurring lipid-soluble organic compounds having as a basis, 17 carbon atoms arranged in four rings and including the sterols (e.g., cholesterol) and sex hormones.

telomere - End region of a chromosome containing characteristic DNA sequences that play an important role in cell division.

tissues - Groups of similar cells organized to carry out one or more specific functions.

toxins - Term applied to poisons in living systems.

Web Resources

Aging/Health/Longevity

http://www.infoplease.com/ipa/A0005140.html

http://pharmrev.aspetjournals.org/content/56/2/163.
long#title7

http://livestrong.com/aboutus/

http://worldhealth.net/

http://go4life.niapublications.org/find-out-about-nia

http://lpi.oregonstate.edu/

Antibiotics

http://inventors.about.com/od/pstartinventions/a/
Penicillin.htm

http://inventors.about.com/od/pstartinventions/a/
Penicillin_2.htm

Bone Health

http://niams.nih.gov/Health_Info/Bone/Osteoporosis/
bone_mass.asp

http://ncbi.nlm.nih.gov/books/NBK38410/

Cancer

http://cancer.org/

http://seer.cancer.gov/statistics/cerquest.org/history-cancer-detection.html

http://nature.com/nrc/journal/v5/n1/fig_tab/nrc1529_I1.html

http://fightaging.org/archives/2001/11/what-is-antiaging.php

http://halls.md/breast/risk.htm

http://nsabp.pitt.edu/

Exercise/Fitness Benefits

http://livestrong.com/article/549070-what-is-supramaximal-exercise/

http://unm.edu/~lkravitz/Article%20folder/epocarticle.html

http://bobdelmonteque.com/

Growth Hormone

http://cedars-sinai.edu/Patients/Health-Conditions/Adult-Growth-Hormone-Deficiency.aspx

Heart Disease

http://heart.org/HEARTORG/

http://framinghamheartstudy.org/about/history.html

Herbal and Plant-Based Supplements

http://supplementquality.com/about.html

http://rain-tree.com/nettles.htm

http://prostate.net/prostate-health-supplements-a-z/
stinging-nettle/

Insulin/Obesity/Dietary Grains/Diabetes

http://news-medical.net/health/Insulin-Resistance-
Pathophysiology.aspx

http://whfoods.org/genpage.php?tname=nutrient&
dbid=111

Miscellaneous

http://library.uchc.edu/departm/hnet/nlist.html

Nutrition

http://urbanext.illinois.edu/veggies/lettuce.cfm

http://cnn.com/2011/health/03/29/grass.grain.
beef.cookinglight/index.html

http://aicr.org/foods-that-fight-cancer/

http://livestrong.com/article/267977-low-glycemic-
nutrition/

http://nutritiondata.self.com/topics/glycemic-index

Oxidative Stress/Antioxidants

http://lpi.oregonstate.edu/

http://lpi.oregonstate.edu/infocenter/phytochemicals/

flavonoids/flavtab2.html

http://cosmosclub.org/web/journals/2002/bulkley.html

http://nutritionadvisor.com/web_md.htm

http://whfoods.org/genpage.php?tname=nutrient&
dbid=111

http://naturalantioxidants.org/

http://naturalantioxidants.org/Total_Antioxidants.html

Plumbing and Sewage

http://theplumber.com/usa.html

http://civil.colorado.edu/~silverst/cven5534/History
%20of%20Wastewater%20Treatment%20in%20
the%20US.pdf

http://sewerhistory.org/articles/whregion/urban_wwm
_mgmt/urban_wwm_mgmt.pdf

Stress/Fatigue/Cortisol/Cortisone

http://biomedcentral.com/1756-0500/4/238

http://cortisolconnection.com/index.php

http://goodtherapy.org/blog/does-perception-stress-
increase-physical-illness-older-adults/

http://dietsinreview.com/diet_column/06/cortisol-the-
stress-hormones-effect-on-your-health-and-weight-loss/
?utm_source=suggested&utm_medium=story&utm_
campaign=outbrain

http://jabfm.org/content/23/2/212.full

Surgery

http://surgery.about.com/od/surgeryinthemedia/a/
   HistoryOfSurgeryTimeline.htm

Sexual Health

http://www2.psych.ubc.ca/~bglab/female.html

http://sexualarousalguide.com/sexual-arousal-
   stimulation-tips.html

http://longevity.about.com/od/lifelongfitness/a
   /exercise_sex.htm

Telomeres/Chromosomes/DNA

http://ch.ic.ac.uk/local/projects/burgoine/origins.txt.html

Testosterone

http://lef.org/magazine/mag2008/dec2008_Destroying-
   the-Myth-about-Testosterone-Replacement-Prostate-
   Cancer_02.htm

Vaccines

http://historyofvaccines.org/content/timelines/all

http://ncbi.nlm.nih.gov/pmc/articles/PMC1200696/
   pdf/bumc0018-0021.pdf

http://historyofvaccines.org/content/timelines/polio

Selected References

Alzheimer's/Cognitive Function

Hormone Replacement Therapy and Cognition. Systematic Review and Meta-analysis Erin S. LeBlanc, Jeri Janowsky, Benjamin K. S., Chan, Heidi D. Nelson. JAMA 2001; 285:1489-1499.

Estrogen Therapy and Cognition: A Review of the Cholinergic Hypothesis Robert B. Gibbs. Endocrine Reviews, April 2010, 31(2):224–253

Estrogen and the Aging Brain: an elixir for the weary cortical network? Dani Dumitriu, Peter Rapp, Bruce McEwen, and John Morrison. Ann N Y Acad Sci. 2010 August ; 1204: 104–112.

Alzheimer's Disease: The Pros and Cons of Pharmaceutical, Nutritional, Botanical, and Stimulatory Therapies, with a Discussion of Treatment Strategies from the Perspective of Patients and Practitioners Wollen, KA. Alt Med Rev 2010; 15 (13): 223-244.

DHA May Prevent Age-Related Dementia Greg M. Cole and Sally A. Frautschy. J. Nutr. 140: 869–874, 2010.

The diagnosis of dementia due to Alzheimer's disease: Recommendations from the National Institute on Aging-Alzheimer's Association workgroups on diagnostic guidelines for Alzheimer's disease Guy M. McKhann et al. Alzheimer's & Dementia (2011); 7: 263–269.

Physical Exercise as a Preventive or Disease-Modifying Treatment of Dementia and Brain Aging J. Eric Ahlskog, Yonas E. Geda, Neill R. Graff-Radford, and Ronald C. Petersen. Mayo Clin. Proc. September 2011; 86(9):876-884

Pharmacology in Health Foods: Effects of Arachidonic Acid and Docosahexaenoic Acid on the Age-Related Decline in Brain and Cardiovascular System Function Yoshinobu Kiso. J Pharmacol Sci 115, 471 – 475 (2011).

Neuroprotective and Ameliorative Actions of Polyunsaturated Fatty Acids Against Neuronal Diseases: Beneficial Effect of Docosahexaenoic Acid on Cognitive Decline in Alzheimer's Disease Michio Hashimoto and Shahdat Hossain. J Pharmacol Sci 115, 471 – 475 (2011).

Timing of Hormone Therapy and Dementia: The Critical Window Theory Re-visited Rachel A. Whitmer, Charles P. Quesenberry Jr, Jufen Zhou, and Kristine Yaffe. Ann Neurol. 2011 January ; 69(1): 163–169.

Calorie Restriction

Calorie Restriction: What Recent Results Suggest for the Future of Aging Research Daniel L. Smith Jr. Tim R. Nagy, David B. Allison. Eur J Clin Invest. 2010 May ; 40(5): 440–450.

Live Better Longer

Dietary Interventions to Extend Life Span and Health Span Based on Calorie Restriction Robin K. Minor, Joanne S. Allard, Caitlin M. Younts, Theresa M. Ward, and Rafael de Cabo. J Gerontol A Biol Sci Med Sci. 2010 July;65(7):695–703

Hormone Replacement Therapy in Women (see also Alzheimer's/Cognition)

Issues to debate on the Women's Health Initiative (WHI) study. Epidemiology or randomized clinical trials - time out for hormone replacement therapy studies? Anette Tùnnes Pedersen and Bent Ottesen. Human Reproduction 2003;18 (11): 2241-2244.

Effects of Conjugated Equine Estrogen in Postmenopausal Women With Hysterectomy The Women's Health Initiative Randomized Controlled Trial. JAMA, April 14, 2004 – Vol 291, No. 14: 1701-1712.

HRT and the Young at Heart (editorial) Michael E. Mendelsohn, M.D., and Richard H. Karas, M.D., Ph.D. NEJM June 21, 2007; 356: 2639-2641.

Conjugated Equine Estrogens and Breast Cancer Risk in the Women's Health Initiative Clinical Trial and Observational Study Ross L. et al. Am J Epidemiol. 2008 June 15; 167(12): 1407–1415.

A Comprehensive Review of the Safety and Efficacy of Bioidentical Hormones for the Management of Menopause and Related Health Risks Deborah Moskowitz, ND. Alternative Medicine Review. 2008; 11 (3): 208-223.

Bioidentical hormones for menopause therapy Cynthia K. Sites. Women's Health 2008; 4(2): 163-171.

Hypogonadism and Testosterone Therapy in Men

Transdermal Testosterone Gel Improves Sexual Function, Mood, Muscle Strength, and Body Composition Parameters in Hypogonadal Men C. Wang et al. The Journal of Clinical Endocrinology & Metabolism. 2000; Vol. 85, No. 8

Diagnosis of Hypogonadism: Clinical Assessments and Laboratory Tests Christina Carnegie. Med Reviews, 2004. 6 (Suppl 6): S3-S8.

Testosterone Replacement in Men With Andropause: An Overview Michael K. Brawer, MD. Rev Urol. 2004;6 (suppl. 6):S9-S15

Hypogonadism in the Man with Erectile Dysfunction: What To Look for and When To Treat Lazarou, S. and Morgantaler, A. Current Urology Reports 2005. 6:476-481.

Endogenous Sex Hormones and Prostate Cancer: A Collaborative Analysis of 18 Prospective Studies Endogenous Hormones and Prostate Cancer Collaborative Group J Natl Cancer Inst 2008;100: 170 – 183

Getting Over Testosterone: Postulating a Fresh Start for Etiologic Studies of Prostate Cancer William R. Carpenter , Whitney R. Robinson , Paul A. Godley. JNCI 2008; 100 (3): 158-159.

Why Is Androgen Replacement in Males Controversial? Glenn R. Cunningham and Shivani M. Toma. J Clin Endocrinol Metab 96: 38–52, 2011

Inflammation – See Also Vascular

Cardiovascular Disease: C-Reactive Protein and the Inflammatory Disease Paradigm: HMG-CoA Reductase Inhibitors, alpha-Tocopherol, Red Yeast Rice, and Olive Oil Polyphenols A Review of the Literature. Lyn Patrick, ND, and Michael Uzick, ND, Lac. Alternative Medicine Review. 2001;6 (3): 248-271.

Diagnostic Implications of C-Reactive Protein Michael A. Zimmerman, MD; Craig H. Selzman, MD; Clay Cothren, MD; Amy C. Sorensen, BS; Christopher D. Raeburn, MD; Alden H. Harken, MD. Arch Surg. 2003;138:220-224

Regulation of survival, proliferation, invasion, angiogenesis, and metastasis of tumor cells through modulation of inflammatory pathways by nutraceuticals Subash C. Gupta, Ji Hye Kim, Sahdeo Prasad, and Bharat B. Aggarwal. Cancer Metastasis Rev. 2010 September ; 29(3): 405–434.

Inflammatory markers in population studies of aging Tushar Singh, MD, MS and Anne B. Newman, MD, MPH. Ageing Res Rev. 2011 July ; 10(3): 319–329.

Association Between High-Sensitivity C-Reactive Protein and Coronary Plaque Subtypes Assessed by 64-Slice Coronary Computed Tomography Angiography in an Asymptomatic Population Jonathan Rubin, MD et al. Circ Cardiovasc Imaging 2011;4;201-209.

Longevity

Search for Mechanisms of Exceptional Human Longevity Natalia S. Gavrilova and Leonid A. Gavrilov. Rejuvenation Research 2010; 13 (2-3): 262-264.

Mammalian models of extended healthy lifespan Colin Selman and Dominic J. Wither. Phil. Trans. R. Soc. B (2011) 366, 99–107.

Oxidative Stress / Antioxidants

Increases in human plasma antioxidant capacity after consumption of controlled diets high in fruit and vegetables Guohua Cao, Sarah L Booth, James A Sadowski, and Ronald L Prior. Am J Clin Nutr 1998;68:1081–7.

Oxidation of Biological Systems: Oxidative Stress Phenomena, Antioxidants, Redox Reactions, and Methods for Their Quantification Ron Kohen and Abraham Nyska. Toxicologic Pathology; 30,(6): 620–650, 2002.

Flavonoid intake and risk of chronic diseases Paul Knekt, Jorma Kumpulainen, Ritva Järvinen, Harri Rissanen, Markku Heliövaara, Antti Reunanen, Timo Hakulinen, and Arpo Aromaa. Am J Clin Nutr. 2002; 76:560–8.

The Antitumor Activities of Flavonoids C. Kanadaswami et al. in vivo 19: 895-910 (2005).

Cruciferous Vegetables and Human Cancer Risk: Epidemiologic Evidence and Mechanistic Basis Jane V. Higdon, Barbara Delage, David E. Williams, and Roderick H. Dashwood. Pharmacol Res. 2007 March ; 55(3): 224–236.

The role of antioxidant supplement in immune system, neoplastic, and neurodegenerative disorders: a point of view for an assessment of the risk/benefit profile Daria Brambilla et al. Nutrition Journal 2008, 7:29.

Antioxidants and Vitamins in Clinical Conditions Z. Zadak et al. Physiol. Res. 58 (Suppl. 1): S13-S17, 2009

Plant polyphenols as dietary antioxidants in human health and disease Kanti Bhooshan Pandey and Syed Ibrahim Rizvi. Oxidative Medicine and Cellular Longevity 2:5, 270-278; November/December; 2009.

Oxidized LDL: Diversity, Patterns of Recognition, and Pathophysiology Irena Levitan, Suncica Volkov, and Papasani V. Subbaiah. Antioxidants & Redox Signaling. 2010; 13 (1): 39-75.

Telomeres

Telomeres and Aging Geraldine Aubert and Peter M. Lansdorp. Physiol Rev 2008; 88: 557–579.

Telomeres and telomerase in cancer Steven E.Artandi_ and Ronald A.DePinho. Carcinogenesis 2010; 31(1):9–18.

Telomere biology in healthy aging and disease Hisko Oeseburg & Rudolf A. de Boer & Wiek H. van Gilst & Pim van der Harst. Eur J Physiol (2010) 459:259–268

The Telomerase Inhibitor Imetelstat Depletes Cancer Stem Cells in Breast and Pancreatic Cancer Cell Lines Immanual Joseph et al. Cancer Res 2010; 70(22); 9494–504.

Human telomerase activity regulation Aneta Wojtyla, Marta Gladych, Blazej Rubis. Mol Biol Rep (2011) 38:3339–3349.

Telomeres in cancer and ageing Luis E. Donate and Maria A. Blasco. Phil. Trans. R. Soc. B (2011) 366, 76–84.

A Natural Product Telomerase Activator as Part of a Health Maintenance Program Calvin B. Harley, Weimin Liu, Maria Blasco, Elsa Vera, William H. Andrews, Laura A. Briggs, and Joseph M. Raffaele. Rejuvenation Research 2011; 14(1): 45-56.

Vascular Disease
(see also Inflammation)

Abdominal Obesity and the Metabolic Syndrome: Contribution to Global Cardiometabolic Risk Jean-Pierre Despre´s, Isabelle Lemieux, Jean Bergeron, Philippe Pibarot, Patrick Mathieu, Eric Larose, Josep Rode´s-Cabau, Olivier F. Bertrand, Paul Poirier. Arterioscler Thromb Vasc Biol 2008; 28:1039-1049.

Periodontal Disease and Coronary Heart Disease Incidence: A Systematic Review and Meta-analysis Linda L. Humphrey, Rongwei Fu, David I. Buckley, Michele Freeman, and Mark Helfand. J Gen Intern Med, 2008; 23(12):2079–86.

Mechanisms of Vascular Aging: New Perspectives Zoltan Ungvari, Gabor Kaley, Rafael de Cabo, William E. Sonntag, and Anna Csiszar. J Gerontol A Biol Sci Med Sci. 2010 October; 65A(10):1028–1041

Live Better Longer

About Hugh Wilson

Dr. Hugh Wilson has been practicing medicine for more than twenty years. He has focused on what causes suffering and death. He has studied how people can alter their lifestyle habits to live a healthier and happier life.

Dr. Wilson completed his undergraduate studies at the University of California, Santa Barbara where he graduated with Highest Honors with a degree in Cell Biology and Physiology. He attended medical school at the University of California, San Francisco. He remained in San Francisco for his post-graduate training where he completed an internship in Internal Medicine at the Pacific Presbyterian Medical Center (now the California Pacific Medical Center). He then took a residency in Anatomic Pathology and Laboratory Medicine also at UCSF.

Dr. Wilson has practiced surgical pathology and laboratory medicine (hematology, immunology, microbiology and clinical chemistry) in Monterey County as well as managing hospital and outpatient medical laboratories, and was certified in Age Management Medicine by the Cenegenics® Education & Research Foundation in 2010.

Live Better Longer

Other Books from Seton Publishing

An award winning veteran broadcast journalist, political consultant, and author, Tony Seton's principal activity over the past two years has been the writing, editing, and publishing of books. They include fiction and non-fiction. Among the recent titles are these:

THE BOY CAPTAIN - Gerard Rose's compelling new historical novel about the early years of a true American hero of the Revolution and the War of 1812.

THE EARLY TROUBLES - Gerard Rose's first historical novel about the Irish struggle for independence during the time of the First World War.

JUST IMAGINE – a scintillating piece of fiction that tells the tell of a man returning from Heaven with a mission to tell Earthlings that they can see auras.

MAYHEM – a contemporary novel set in Marin County, California based on the mythic struggle between good and evil, with the author being called in to tip the tide of the titanic battle.

THE AUTOBIOGRAPHY OF JOHN DOUGH, GIGOLO – a novel about a former hedge fund manager who decides on a new path – to improve the lives of women. His clients include widows, divorcees and a gangster's moll.

SILVER LINING – a novel about a shooting on the street that brings reporter David Skye and nurse Lucy Balfour together, for what becomes excitement and romance.

THE OMEGA CRYSTAL – a page-turner of a novel about how the oil industry is sitting on crucial developments in solar power waiting until their inventories run dry.

TRUTH BE TOLD – a novelized version of a true story about an historic civil rights case of sexual harassment against a top-50 American law school.

THE QUALITY INTERVIEW / GETTING IT RIGHT ON BOTH SIDES OF THE MIC – a guide of interviewing for interviewers and interviewees of every stripe.

FROM TERROR TO TRIUMPH / THE HERMA SMITH CURTIS STORY – a true story of a young girl's survival of the Nazi occupation of Austria and her creation of a successful new life on the Monterey Peninsula.

THE SHADOW CANDIDATE – a compelling political novel written by veteran consultant Rich Robinson who gets unerringly close to the truth about politics today.

VISION FOR A HEALTHY CALIFORNIA – a road map for the Golden State, written by Bill Monning, the highly-esteemed member of the California Assembly.

THREE LIVES OF A WARRIOR – the stunning memoir of Phil Butler, who spent eight years as a prisoner of the North Vietnamese and came home to a new life.

If you are interested in these books, or in having your own book written, edited and/or published, please go online to SetonPublishing.com.